THRIVE *Again*

Simple Strategies to Time Out, Tune In and Tone Up Your Life

THRIVE*Again*

Simple Strategies to Time Out, Tune In and Tone Up Your Life

ISBN 978-0-692-56796-8

Printed in the United States of America.

All photography by: www.TreySingleton.com

THRIVE *Again*

Simple Strategies to Time Out, Tune In and Tone Up, Your Life

Eli de Moraes, M.A.,M.F.A., R.Y.T.

© Kaizen Phoenix Publishing

DEDICATION

~~~

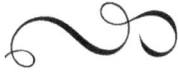

My husband, Andre.

Thank you for believing in me before I believed in myself. You never falter in your belief or dedication to our family and me, and for that we are deeply blessed. I love you.

Our girls, Helena and Isabella

You both are my inspiration to live a big and bold life. It is my dream and mission to live fully and reach high, so to be a shining example that anything is possible for you. You both are going to make powerful and positive impacts on the world! *In my heart!*

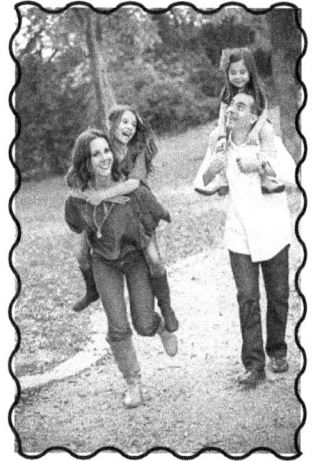

to **YOU**

This book is also dedicated to all of you hard working, amazing women who know they were placed on this earth to make a difference. May you always take a stand to live your authentic self, by caring fully for yourself and living healthfully and purposefully on your terms. Only then can you fully express yourself and THRIVE Again!

CONTENTS

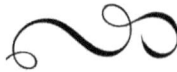

Part IV

Tone Up Your Body and Mind Through Food, Movement,
Mindfulness and Relaxation!

ACKNOWLEDGEMENTS

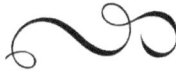

I must first thank God for placing me on this earth to live my life fully. Only through Him can I live the life for which He created me. With all my heart, I know that He placed me and YOU here on this planet at this time in history to make a difference and it is only by getting out of the way of ourselves, plus nurturing ourselves along the way, that this can happen. He has placed a big vision in my heart and this book is just a small step toward greater things He has planned. My prayer is that I open myself up enough to act as a vessel for His message about the importance of getting back to our core and nurturing it.

To my husband. Thank you for never wavering in your support in EVERYTHING I do. You are my husband, best friend, lover and confidant. Your words of: "You don't have a right to question yourself and your God-given gifts!" will forever ring in my heart. I love you.

To our girls, Helena and Isabella. You are my angels. You are two big reasons I keep breathing and my heart keeps beating. I thank you for your patience as I pushed through this book and learned to trust in myself. You both have been two of my biggest teachers in life and it is my prayer that I live as fully as I can, pushing through doubts and fears, so to give you proof ANYTHING is possible if you set your dreams into action.

To my parents. Huh, where do I begin? As a family of three, no matter what heavy challenges came our way as I was growing up, I ALWAYS knew

I was loved and supported to see my dreams to reality. As scientists you probably had no clue how to guide this artist into a career, but still you did it. When I said I wanted to go off on my own and move to Europe to dance, choreograph and teach, you said "OK, go for it!" You always had full trust in me and my abilities as I tried to figure it all out. You have always been a constant source of strength and love in my life and I would not be the person I am today had it not been for you, your love and your sacrifice. I love you thiiiiiiiis big!

To my past and present clients. I think you truly bless me more than what I provide you! Because of you I am able to live out my purpose and passion and for that I am deeply grateful. April, Suzanne, Lindy, Summer, Susan, Tay, Christi, Donna, Haley, Patricia, Krista, Juliana, Toni, Teri, and Stephanie, this book has been birthed through the work we have been doing together this year. You are big inspirations for this book.

I want to give an extra acknowledgment to Tay Devereaux-Hutchison and Christi Greene for the development of this book. You both have truly helped me flesh out my ideas through letting me talk things through as well as provide helpful insight into the lives of many women. Your honesty, insight and integrity are en pointe and real. You rock!

To Krista Murry. Thank you for your expertise and talent in designing the inner workings of this book! Your eye and creativity is a God-given talent and I deeply appreciate you sharing it here.

To my friends, colleagues, mastermind partners (Susie, Darla and Susanna), and my queenly Divine Living Academy sisters: All I can say is that each of you is my inspiration, and for that, I am deeply and forever blessed. Through the manner in which you live your lives, I can see what great impact we can all make in the world when we, 1. truly live life on purpose as our authentic selves, 2. let go of self-limiting beliefs, 3. step out to be fully visible, 4. create a plan in line with one's vision, and 5. GET INTO INSPIRED ACTION! You are my (s)heros! I love you!

And to my coaches at:

Eli de Moraes

The Institute of Integrative Nutrition, both for Health Coaching and through the Launch Your Dream Book Course. Joshua Rosenthal, Lindsey Smith, Patty Bean, Sue Brown, Marie Ann Mosher, Kathleen B. Norris, Mariss Leigh, and Kathleen DiChiara, all I can say is that every element of this institution and your leadership have rocked my world. You truly are making waves that are being felt throughout the world. Thank you. Thank you. Thank you.

And to my queenly coaches of the Divine Living Academy, Gina Devee, Megan Huber, Giovanna Capozza, and Julia Evans. You have shown me that ANYTHING is possible. And this is only the beginning! THANK YOU!

I would be remiss if I did not say thank you to my fabulous photographer, Trey Singleton, of www.TreySingleton.com. His creative eye is magic and he was able to nail my idea of the whole look I envisioned! Thank you, Trey!

INTRODUCTION

We're On the Crazy-Busy Bus

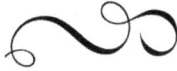

When am I going to learn I can't do it all?!? I never have enough time, am crazy-busy and have to be so many things for so many people. If someone else wants a piece of me I will explode!

This is a text I recently received from a client who had found herself completely out of sorts and overwhelmed while trying to juggle a full time career, a husband and her precious young children. She was at wits' end and knew she needed to somehow create boundaries in her life. She had placed her foot heavily on the acceleration pedal while driving what I call the 'Crazy-Busy Bus' and needed to get off! But how? This is the million dollar question!

In this day and age, we can easily get profoundly busy with the multitude of responsibilities we take on, along with all the other attention grabbing pulls and distractions in our modern society. We, as women, for some reason, also tend to place huge expectations upon ourselves and raise the bar of ultimate perfectionism to being able to do EVERYTHING. In doing so, we ultimately set ourselves up for failure because we realistically cannot get everything on our "TO-DO" list accomplished in the way we feel we should by day's end. We easily lose sight of the connection to our lives, priorities, and bodies and wonder where the hell we went. Our life begins living us instead of us living it. We cannot get off the hamster wheel, with the result of feeling sick of only surviving through life.

Sound familiar? Are you driving your own Crazy-Busy Bus? I know I can still easily find myself lead-footing mine (I have named my bus, Fred) if I am not careful.

A few years ago, I had a very successful business in which I lived, breathed and slept work, all in the name of giving my family a bigger and better shot in life. Long story short, I was so highly driven on building my business, along with taking care of my small family, that I had resorted to sleeping and eating very little. My husband joked that I could live off of air, but I felt I was strong enough, could push through, and was invincible. Little did I know. I knew the vitamins my company sold were good, so my conclusion was that I must be getting the nutrients I needed, and thus believed it was OK to sleep very few hours and forget to eat. Yes, you just heard that from a Health Coach who is a big proponent of eating real and good food, and sleeping a full night, but we all have to come from somewhere, right!?

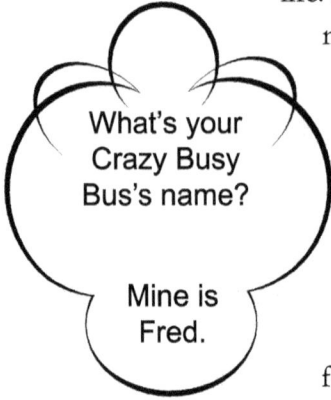

What's your Crazy Busy Bus's name?

Mine is Fred.

In the middle of it, my husband was laid off, which put me in total survival mode to make this business work. I was living in a constant 'fight or flight' state, never allowing myself down time. 'Me' time was non-existent and a luxury I never thought I could afford, let alone deserved.

One night my husband found me on the ground in our backyard, wrapped in a blanket having a nervous breakdown. I had become addicted to being busy as well as the adrenaline that came from constantly living in that mode of 'fight or flight'. To keep that adrenaline flowing I had to reach an even greater amount of stress to get my 'hit'. I crashed. I took my busy-ness as a sign to myself and others that I was successful and had value. **I wore my exhaustion as a badge of honor**, thinking that I was proving that I was positively contributing to the world. What resulted was a broken woman, an empty wreck with adrenal fatigue, a leaky gut (small tears in the intestine caused by stress, allowing larger-than-needed food particles into the blood stream), thinning hair, and depression like no one's business.

Eli de Moraes

I knew things had to change. I lived 'shoulding' all over myself...*I should be doing this. I should be doing that. I should be better than that.* was a constant recording that played in my head. Things needed to change. And they did. Fortunately, for the better.

I slowly learned that, at the fundamental core of life, I had and have to live fully nurturing myself, FIRST. I was able, with diet change and supplement therapy, heal my leaky gut. I learned to meditate and slow my mind, so that I could focus better. Through various stress management tools, I learned how to better deal with stressors, or not allow them to affect me at all. I also learned that eating whole, real foods and making sleep a sacred act of living, rather something I fit in because I just had to, could change everything for my health. Most importantly, I learned that if I do not put myself first (after God), before all people and situations that come up, I will not be able to serve and love those who I cherish the most. **THIS was the game-changer**.

Looking back, I see that I experienced this period of turmoil and triumph so to be able to teach and guide others how to do the same. We live in a world that appears to be addicted to constant motion and action, rather than enjoying being still at times. I know I am not the only one who stresses over life. And I would be lying if I said I don't fall victim to stressors even after the work I have done that I outline in this book.

Now I just have more awareness to rein myself back with more conscious choices and behaviors. I still sometimes allow things to get overscheduled, thinking I can get the kids to school, pick up the dog from the groomer, pick up those much needed eggs for a meal later in the day, get the mail and pick up the house before a client comes over. All. In . The . Course . Of . Thirty . Minutes! Yeah, right, Wonder Woman, that's not going to fly!

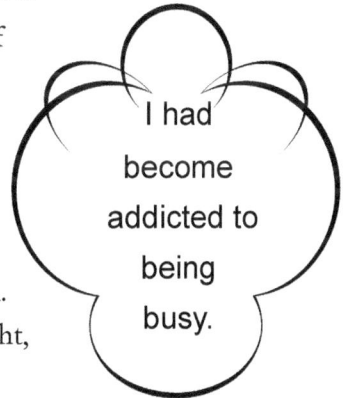

I had become addicted to being busy.

If I am not careful, I can also create more stress, internally. I can worry about our kids. I have fears of failing *and* succeeding. I stress over finances. I can find myself placing unnecessary anxiety on myself of not being good enough at endeavors I attempt. Our family still lives with an undercurrent of fear of my husband getting laid off again. It is after all Corporate America, and those literal knee-buckling calls from him stating his department had been closed, the company had down-sized, and that he was coming home mid-day, still can make my stomach jump at any remark of things potentially going sour at his current job. What I am saying is that I am not immune, but I now have tools to get out of it and look forward to sharing them with you!

Fortunately, what I found is that most of the changes we have to make to ease our foot off the stress pedal are actually simple and fun.

So, before we get started, let me remind you of something. NO ONE like you has EVER existed in the history of all humankind! Never has the exact combination of cells in a person's body formed into someone like you. No one has ever had the same combination of life experiences that you have had. What this means is that no one can predict what amazing things you can accomplish in your lifetime if you ease yourself off of being stressed all the time! Your past does not determine your present or your future. No one is holding you back, except possibly yourself. If you are in overload, it's time to reframe your inner recordings of your life stories from ones of perceived failure, mistakes, and struggle, to those of insight, breakthroughs, and growth opportunities. It's time to learn to shed the need to constantly fill your schedule to stay busy, for whatever reasons you might have, so to thrive in the life you were placed here to live.

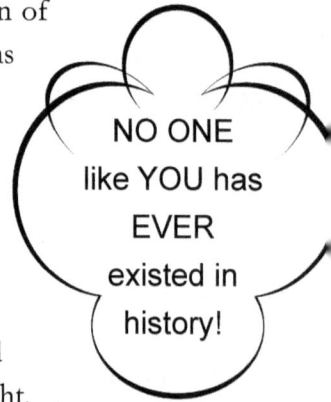

NO ONE like YOU has EVER existed in history!

Let's make a deal, alright? No longer do you have time, or are available, to be the driver of your "Crazy-Busy Bus". It's time to understand the non-negotiable mindset that it is your total responsibility to take care of yourself, first, mentally, physically and spiritually, before all else. I know this can be a difficult one to swallow, but I have to give you the hard truth that if you are not taking care of yourself the way you need, you are not doing as much good for your family, work, and community as you hope. Just think about the example you are giving your kids (if you have them) if you are constantly running, full of anxiety, overscheduled, and busy. Is that the legacy you want to leave them with to repeat in their lives? I doubt it.

Let's also make another deal. Please stop running after things that give you anxiety because of your perception of other people's expectations of you. I promise that when you do, such freedom and peace will fall upon you, affecting all those around you. Remember, you are not responsible for everyone else's actions, happiness, and attitudes. It is OK to say no to people and requests if they do not support your long-term well-being, life goals and values. Remember that life is truly too long to live in agony and too short to waste it. You were created to inspire the world in your own way and being constantly busy ain't gonna get you there! No apologies required.

Through the reading of this book, it is my hope that you walk away feeling more peace, joy, and health in your life and feel more grounded. I expect you to:

- Develop an understanding of what causes stress and the detrimental aspects it has on your overall health, weight management, and well-being

- Understand stress management vs. stress prevention. I have spent years in the profession of stress management as a certified and registered personal trainer, yoga/meditation and Pilates instructor, but what I find is that if we do not address the causes of stress in our lives, any type of 'management' is temporary and unsustainable. Let's get to the bottom of our stress and nip it in the bud!

- Pinpoint and develop your top priorities in life and then stay focused on them through your actions

- Become more aware of how to respond to and prevent your stress triggers and gain tools on how to take positive actions that best support your needs when stress does hit. Some include more productive scheduling practices that match your priorities, eating better, creating better sleep patterns and rituals, to name a few.

- Become more confident in your decisions around the boundaries you create

- 'Arm' yourself with self-supporting techniques to keep you in check and allow your new lifestyle to be sustainable

- Become trusting that you can be more productive by doing less. It's OK, and actually imperative to your survival to literally sit and be still, mentally, physically, and spiritually. You will also live more in the present moment, rather than so much in the past and future.

- Learn ways in which to create personal down, or 'me' time, with more mindfulness, even when you feel you have no time. You will also learn to embrace the notion that down time is non-negotiable and a priority, not a guilty pleasure or luxury.

- Very importantly, you will take ownership of your life instead of feeling like a victim to it living you! There is no more sacrificing your health and well-being for your version of success.

- And finally, you will become more dynamically balanced (we will discuss what this is in more detail later) concerning the support systems you need in place when life gets more intense. As a result, you will be able to handle those inevitable crazy days with ease and more energy to make a greater impact in your lifetime.

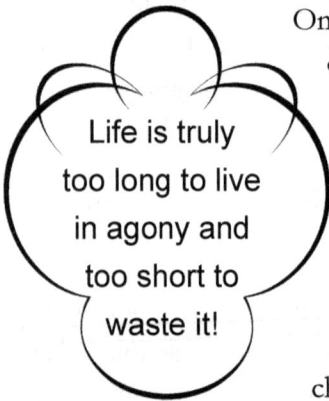

One word of warning: as you go through this process of becoming aware, clearing, letting go, and creating new modes of living for yourself, please know that at times you may feel like a fish out of water. If you do, just keep pushing forward because you will soon see the results.

Life is truly too long to live in agony and too short to waste it!

Let me give you an example. One of my responsibilities as a Pilates teacher is to help my clients correct their posture. When I show them the correct placement they inevitably tell me they are crooked. I know they are in alignment as all joints and body parts are where they should be for optimal functioning, but because the person has been operating in an imbalanced manner for so long, the correct way feels wrong and foreign. Once you trust that another way creates more freedom and then develop strength around it, you begin to thrive more. I invite you to see this process in the same way. You may feel off, or awkward, but in time, you will find your life naturally flowing more fluidly!

Another warning: no matter how much work you do through this book you will still have days that get crazy because so many unexpected things happen that are out of your control. Give yourself grace and remember the tools you learn here. The systems you put in place will help you make it through.

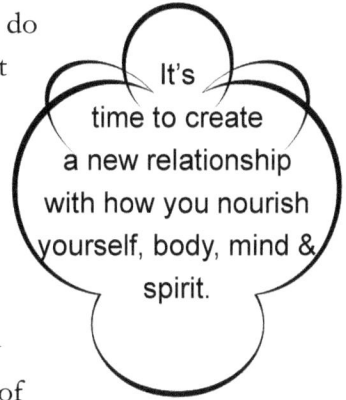

It's time to create a new relationship with how you nourish yourself, body, mind & spirit.

Every single living being is inspired to continually expand and grow. Given the right nutrients, a blade of grass, for example, will effortlessly continue to reach for the sky. If a rock or a branch gets in its way, it simply moves around it and keeps moving and reaching. This is the essence of life. When a living being is functioning, fully supported by what it needs to thrive, it continues to live effortlessly and ever-expansive. You are meant to live like this, too! By giving yourself the right foods, the environment, the right mindset and movement, you will be able to function in your best place.

Please know that I have felt and experienced every aspect of what I speak about in this book: stress, anxiety, being overwhelmed, lack of sleep, interrupted sleep, excessive clutter, Super Woman complex, bad food habits, over-eating, under eating, messed up hormones, guilt over not doing enough, crazy thyroid, heart palpitations, depression, feeling like I am not enough, messed up fitness regimens, and so much more. You name it, I probably had it or did it.

You may currently be in a completely different place in life than what I just described with things going pretty well. There might be areas of the book that do not relate to you, so skip those. You may pick this up at another point in your life and need every aspect of it. Use this book for what you need it. Take and leave what works best for you. But if you find you are really feeling like something has to change, then follow as many of the pointers as possible.

I am continually told I now make living vibrantly and healthfully look effortless. My life is not perfect, but it IS easier if you put in the hard work like I have and still do. I work toward setting and sticking with my priorities and boundaries. I also work at clearing unnecessary stresses and effectively addressing stresses when they come. I also strive to move, and feed my body, mind and spirit with the most life-giving energy I can find. My goal is to teach you to do the same.

I have practiced every exercise in this book and still integrate them daily. I assure you that they work, if you work the plan. And only if you work the plan. I know you can too, and turn your life around and THRIVE AGAIN just like I have! **No longer are you available to be in the state where all you do is prep to fully live!**

I invite you to take a stand for your life, starting from the inside out. Begin to have a new relationship with how you nourish yourself, body, mind and spirit. So let's go time out, tune in, and tone up!!! It's time to create a #newnormal!

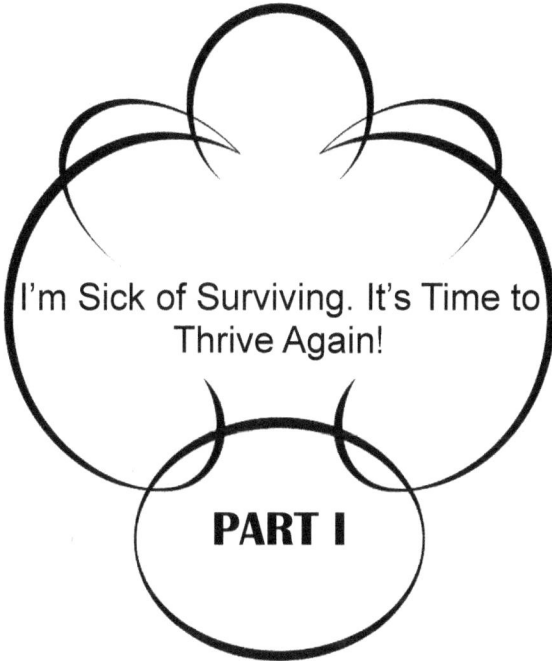

I'm Sick of Surviving. It's Time to Thrive Again!

PART I

CHAPTER ONE

Stress and Its Chokehold On Our Body, Mind and Spirit

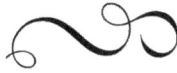

Tension is who you think you should be. Relaxation is who you are.
Chinese Proverb

Where are we getting all this stress and the incessant need to be busy? How can we prevent stress in the first place and manage it when it hits?

First, it is important to understand what excessive stress can do to our bodies so that we have a reason to even address it. We need to take a quick look at our actual nervous system and how our bodies are meant to respond to life's stresses.

While growing up, I heard that stress is one of the leading causes of chronic illness, such as heart disease, cancer, and diabetes. It is also found to cause us to have a higher risk of depression, auto-immune disorders, decreased brain size, high cholesterol, increased fat stores, loss of libido, stroke, premature aging, and hyper tension, to name a few. I originally thought that the notion that stress increased your risk of disease was crazy. I naïvely responded with the thought that you should just not have stress in your life! Ha! Little did I know that it is not that easy and that my passion later in life would be to help people lessen that stress in their lives! I didn't quite understand how that could be until I started experiencing stress myself.

Can you believe that according to the CDC, more than 75% of medical costs in our country are from chronic diseases that are stress related? When I hear this, it makes me even more determined to get the word out on how imperative it is to prevent and manage our stress. This means that we have to become aware and put our foot down, stating that enough is enough. Change can be difficult, especially when it comes to lifestyle and what is seen as against the norm of society. However, if you believe it will make things better for your life, change is much easier than the turmoil, high expense, anxiety and tragedy that come with ill health. I don't know about you, but I don't want my husband missing his wife and kids missing their mommy because she died from self-inflicted stress! What this means is two things:

I know I can easily feel the zombie-pull toward the blue screen in the wee hours of the morning (and night!)

• We need to learn how to decrease what we allow into our lives and schedules.

• And we need to learn how to more mindfully deal with stress. We must gain the ability to more effectively and quickly get back to the state of equilibrium our bodies need to rest and heal. Chaotic mind = chaotic life and ill body. Calm mind = calmer life and healthier body.

Just like the heart is meant to contract AND release so to effectively pump blood, our entire being (body, mind and spirit) needs to release and relax. We have become incredibly detached from the true needs of our bodies, thinking that we can push them harder, faster and longer without ramifications, and then wonder why we are exhausted, fatigued, irritable, and developing expensive chronic diseases. The body will ALWAYS present its bill if you do not respect and nurture it properly.

But I digress. Back to the science-y part…

Basically, our nervous system is made up of our sympathetic and para-sympathetic systems. The sympathetic aspect is what we are more conscious of, including our actions and reactions. This is also where the 'fight or flight' mechanism comes into play. Back when we lived on the land and in caves, we had lions and tigers and bears, oh, my! (Sorry, I couldn't resist!) When

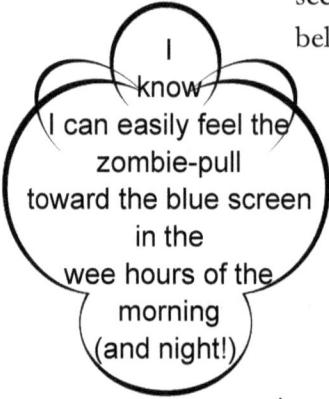

we came upon a danger, our adrenaline and cortisol got cranked up, so that we could more powerfully either fight said animal or run like a bat out of hell to get away. The same holds true now when a perceived threat looms. This is the alarm state where we go into panic mode to protect ourselves. Our pulse, blood pressure, blood sugar, fats, and respiration increase and the pupils dilate. Everything goes to survival mode.

Once the perceived, or actual, danger is gone, our parasympathetic system kicks into play. This system is what regulates everything in our body we don't have to consciously think about to keep us alive. It is what regulates our heart to pump, our breathing, and all other functions in our body. It is also known as the 'rest and digest' aspect of our existence. Once the parasympathetic system gets to play and be on the forefront, our body becomes more even-keeled and more at peace.

Our breathing becomes regular with more 'belly', or diaphragmatic breathing, instead of upper chest breathing. We are more relaxed and our bodies can more effectively digest and rest/sleep so to recuperate and heal from the day's stresses. In so doing, the body can be strong for the next time we come upon another life-threatening danger.

This is the state where we need to be most of the time for optimal health, with an occasional kick of adrenaline to get things accomplished. A little stress is good and needed.

Remember, you are NOT responsible for everyone else's actions, happiness, & attitudes.

Unfortunately, our perception of what an emergency is has become skewed and our 'fight or flight' mode has become a habit. Because of all the information coming at us as well as technology that we have incorporated into our lives to supposedly make life more streamlined, non-life threatening situations have become our proverbial 'tigers' and 'bears.' We feel we can, and must, stuff more in to keep up and thus, get frantic.

High work demands, emails, cell phone calls, daily commutes, all our kids' activities, texts, Facebook, work, voicemails, cooking, fear of job loss, instant

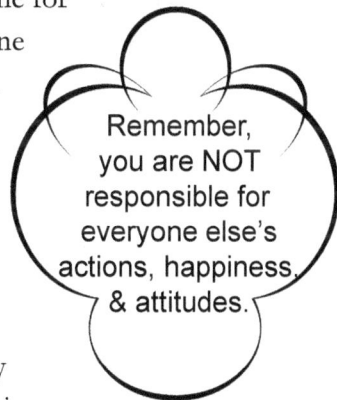

messages, debt, computer glitches, 24/7 newscasts and much more are now our perceived emergencies.

We also easily inject more background noise into our lives than needed (like volunteering for everything asked of us, overscheduling everyone in the family, watching an excess of TV and technology, etc.), and, as a result, can feel overwhelmed and fatigued. On top of it, we feel we have no time to really cook homemade meals, so easily resort to pre-made, processed, under-nourishing fast food alternatives.

To compensate that fatigue, we then drink our coffee to trick our bodies into the feeling we can do more and, as a result, push harder to get *just one more thing in*! Instead, we should be drinking more water, eating real foods and getting to bed earlier, but the temptation to finally get things done once the house is calm in the evening pulls on us to push deep into the night, making us more and more sleep deprived. I know not putting so much on our plates is so much easier said than done. We don't have time, or cannot afford to chill out and just 'be', right?!

Be honest. How often do you start your day with time-sucking temptations of checking emails and Facebook before you even get out of bed? Pinterest? Instagram? I know I can easily feel the zombie-pull toward the blue screen in the wee hours of the morning (and night!). How about being tempted to answer every call that comes in, or respond to every text, even when you are in the middle of something more important with other people?

How about the incessant habit of checking your phone every time you stop at a red light? In doing so, we never stay focused on one thing, causing us, in turn, to think we have ADD and memory loss! The main problem is that we are on information overload and don't stay focused on the task, or people at hand! We have easily become addicted to gaining more and more information. No brain is meant to do so many quick-shifting things at one time!

And you moms out there. How often do you get the kids down and feel like you can finally get everything you need to get done now that is it quiet? Laundry, balancing the budget, study, work on your business, clean the house, etc., etc., etc.. If you do this (here's another bit of science!), **your**

cortisol levels will start rising again when they are meant to be dropping in order to get a full night of deep rest. This might also contribute to your weight gain around your belly. For all you self-professed Night Owls, this means that because you keep pushing when you should be closing down your day, you get a spike in energy. You can probably get to sleep when you finally lie down, but then keep waking up through the night because of a disruption in hormones, like your cortisol.

Been there, done that. I promise you, if you shift your mind set, start listening to your natural body cycles, along with the cycles of nature, and wake early to get all that done, instead of staying up late, you will see a HUGE change in how you get things done and how your body feels. It is truly amazing.

> Just like the heart, our entire being (body, mind and spirit) needs to contract AND relax.

Getting back to this 'fight or flight' state that I mentioned … if we get caught in a loop and, more often than not, live in this mode, we go into what is called the adaptive state. Here, we constantly barrage the body with adrenaline and other chemicals and hormones. When this happens, the body becomes resistant to going back to that more stable state governed by your parasympathetic system. We, in a sense, become addicted to the adrenaline, making it more difficult to access the 'rest and digest' state, causing us to be more susceptible to illness due to a suppressed immune system. We also can more easily pack on the pounds that seem so resistant to be lost.

So, instead of simply getting back to our natural state of balance through doing less and focusing on true rest, we think that all the side effects of our stressful lives need to be 'fixed' with more activity. We pile on more 'to-do's', work out harder, and drink more caffeine to keep moving. No wonder we are so tired and down on ourselves. If we could just trust that just 'being' every once in a while is enough, much of the anxiety in our lives would seriously slough off and out of our lives!

Now, if we are in this heightened adaptive state for too long, we hit the exhaustion stage. This is where all bodily resources are depleted and the body,

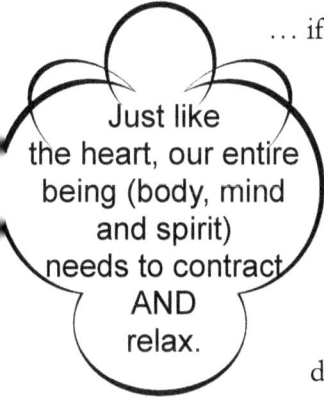

mind, and spirit go into burn-out mode. We crash and burn. This is what I hit when found wrapped in my blanket that fateful night and where so many others of you might find yourself today.

It's time to somehow stop this never-ending cycle! We are getting sicker, fatter, more fatigued, and irritable and never feel like we can get it all done … all for the sake of … what? If we can get in alignment with all parts of our lives, our health and well-being naturally come back.

Below I invite your to list out all the things you are currently stressing over. What is causing you to stay on your Crazy-Busy Bus? List them, doodle them, whatever works for you!

Also, think about and make notes on where you stand in relation to your health around: family, recreation, travel, adventure, spiritual practice, cooking, eating, relaxation, relationships/romance, career, etc.. Get a notebook if you feel you need more space, as you will be writing more throughout the book.

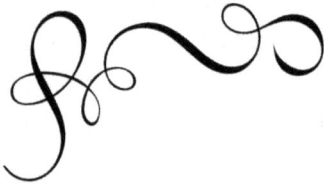

TIME OUT THOUGHTS

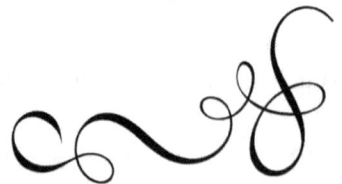

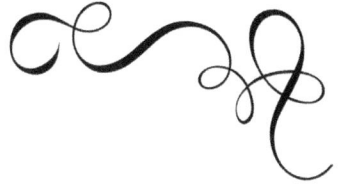

If you are reading an electronic version of his book, please get a notebook for your notes and thoughts. Let the outside be a reflection of you. You may want to get one even if you have the hard copy so that you feel more spacious with your thoughts.

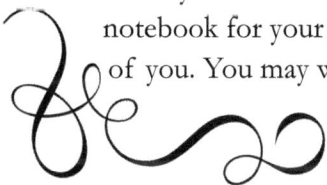

CHAPTER TWO

Let's Get Off The Crazy-Busy Bus!

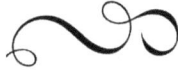

I mentioned it earlier and we made a deal, but let's talk about it again. Change can be simple, yet difficult to implement. It's time for a come-to-Jesus meeting, my friend.

I know. We, as women, want to contribute to the world as well as often contribute to our family's income by following a career. We also tend to take it upon ourselves to be the caregivers, cooks, event planners, social calendar coordinators, taxi drivers and sex goddesses in the bedroom. We can easily feel we are doing it ALL while living right on the edge of screaming: "IF SOMEONE ELSE WANTS A PIECE OF ME, I MIGHT EXPLODE!" We can easily feel we are being lived, rather than us living our lives the way God intended them to be lived. We can feel lost in the middle of it. I seriously do not think I can count on one hand the number of women in my life who feel balanced and in control of their lives and schedules.

I also know that many of us walk around wearing the 'crazy-busy' as a badge of honor. We are the queens of multi-tasking. Hey, didn't our generation coin the term? **We tend to gain value by being busy and keeping up with all the juggling of everything we take on.** It seems as if the one who takes on the most, volunteers the most, takes the kids to the most activities, all while looking amazing, is the winner. I have to tell you that that 'winner' is probably crumbling inside! Her crazy bus is likely caroming out of control, about to lose a wheel.

My friend, it's time to stop the madness! Let's get real and turn the light back on ourselves for a good view. We need to expose how we are actually creating ALL of this and placing it on ourselves by the way we respond to external pulls and internal expectations. Let's release the chokehold we have on our lives and get off the hamster wheel. We are so afraid to stop because our world might fall apart.

Are we just adding more to our plates because we can? What truly lies under the need to keep busy? Are we afraid of the silence that resting brings? It's time to simplify and shed the mental and physical crap in our lives so to live a life that oozes health and vitality.

Balance is a choice. And I am not talking about the balance that is static where all-parts-of-your-life-are-well-and-perfect, kind of balance. I am talking about what I call **dynamic balance**. This is where there is a constant shifting and choosing of responses to what comes your way. This is not about being in control of everything, but how we oversee and respond to those things we influence, informed by our priorities. By choice. Not by default. We can choose to go way off center during certain life events or to accomplish particular projects, but we must have the plan, or 'tethers' in our mind as to how and when we will readjust back the other way. **We have to remember that we can do anything, but not everything.**

Everything you do and how you respond to your life is YOUR CHOICE. What you schedule is your choice. How much sleep you get is your choice. What and who you allow in your environment is your choice. Yes, there are some things that affect us that initially feel out of our control, but what we do with that information is up to us. If we are not sleeping through the night, maybe it is because our hormones are off. If so, it is up to us to get them looked at. When we truly take this concept to heart, we fully take responsibility for our life. It will no longer live us.

Now, I do need to say a quick side note about depression, in relation to our choices. If you suffer, or if you ever have suffered from it, you know it is not something you can just snap out of. If one could, one would, right? There is not much out there that can be lonelier or emotionally and physically painful as depression. If you do suffer from it, give yourself space and grace. Address the depression head on as soon as you realize you have it. Get support, get blood work done and nurture yourself. Just like weight loss, it is not about willpower. Systems (hormones, chemicals, micro-nutrients) could be ever so slightly off and wreak havoc on your mental and emotional states. Dig deep, get answers and get well. Once you do, you will have so much more clarity and energy to attack this book!

We can truly choose our pace and not be swept up by all the external forces that may come our way. When we take hold of our choices, aligned with our priorities, we become better humans, wives, mothers, friends and co-workers. We are more able to make the impact we want to make, whether as hard working employees, moms, entrepreneurs, world stage influencers, or all of the above!

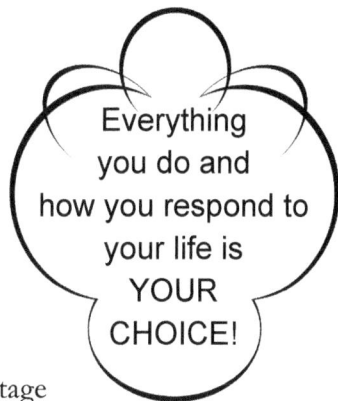

Everything you do and how you respond to your life is YOUR CHOICE!

It's time to have more by having and doing less: more fun, more moving, more music, more prayer, and more abundance. We can do this by having less 'stuff' in our lives that we have to be in charge of. Declutter every aspect of your life, from your physical and electronic 'piles', junk mail and requests from others, to your closet, calendar and mind. When we do this we give ourselves more space to truly enjoy our lives on our terms.

Allow yourself to forgive yourself of anything you might have done in the past that keeps you in the busy mode. You are and always have been enough and are a constant work in progress. Every bit of wisdom you need is inside of you, if you trust it.

Now, FULLY trust me when I say that it is imperative that you start living your life focused on taking care of YOU, FIRST. There are no ifs, ands, or buts here. There is no more going back to always putting yourself last.

As a result, you will feel more at ease, rested, healthier, and possibly weighing less, all while the rest of your family learns from your example. They, in turn, will feel less stress, be healthier and more connected to you *and* each other. If you are there for yourself, you can be more present and better prepared to care for them with even more love and nourishment. Win. Win. Win!

Before we move into the action part of this book, I invite you to take a moment to pause. **Pause and take a breath. A deep breath.** A few deep breaths. Feel all the sweetness of life enter your being like you are inhaling the scent of your favorite home-cooked baked treat someone special made for you. Relish it. How do you feel? Joyful? Taken care of? Loved? At peace? You can always return to this place at any time!

If you are the praying type, pray that this journey you are commencing for yourself and all those around you be prospered by God, or your higher power. Ask that He/She guide your every step of the way toward healing and THRIVING; a thriving life HE created you to have! Expect super natural blessings to occur! Ask for the ideal life that you desire that is more dynamically balanced. Now have faith and trust, with peace, that it will happen.

You might find it a little strange, but I like to compare praying and the faithful trust needed that it will come to that of ordering at a restaurant. When we place our order at a restaurant we fully trust it will come eventually, right? We don't doubt it. We go about enjoying and being active, but trust our nourishment will come soon. I invite you do the same here. Trust that He is ready to provide, if you are ready to receive, nourishment for your mind, body and spirit! What is profound is that when you open yourself up to listening and receiving, by working through the exercises in this book, He will show you the life He wants you to have. He wouldn't have placed your desires in your heart if He didn't fully want them for you. He will also provide all provisions to attain those desires. So just listen, receive and get into action.

Are we just adding more to our plates because we can?

The remainder of the book is all about you and your process! Trust it and yourself. See it as sort of a workbook for you to walk through with simple tasks that can offer you profound results toward a thriving life.

Let's accomplish more by doing less! How about more 'being' and less 'doing', so that you can truly be present for the precious moments in your life?

Let's time out, tune in, and tone up!

Write any notes you might like to write, or doodle before we get started.

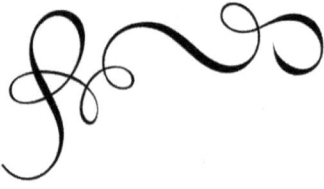

It always seems impossible until it's done! –Nelson Mandela.

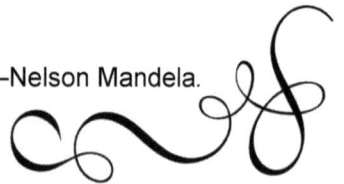

Eli de Moraes

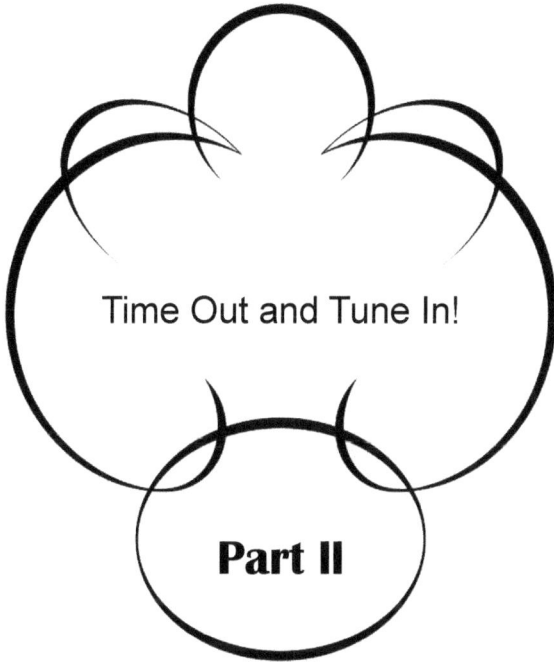

Time Out and Tune In!

Part II

CHAPTER THREE

Your Big Vision and Prioritize, Prioritize, Prioritize

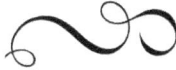

Don't be pushed by your problems, but led by your dreams.
Ralph Waldo Emerson

As we enter the fun action part of the book, I have one rule. NO MULTI-TASKING! **Focus here and in the now!** Agreed? Good!

Now is the time to truly gift yourself the gift of timing out and tuning in to what you envision your healthy thriving life will look like. Go get yourself your favorite blanket, a cup of tea, or glass of wine (my choice!) and take some time to nourish yourself, body, mind and spirit. Set a date with yourself and focus.

Now that we have that clear, I invite you to ask yourself two things. If you do not answer these (especially the second one) and tackle them head on, I assure you that you will not see this entire process through. Truly take time in the space provided to write out, draw, or cut and paste pictures. You can even move those to a large poster board and create a beautiful Vision Board to put up for you to see on an ongoing basis to keep you on track. Doing so will probably be more impactful for you.

Use whatever medium works best for you. I am a visual person, so magazine cutouts put on a poster board works best for me. For you, you might rather write it all out. Doing both might even be better! Now, go!

THRIVE*Again*

Let's visualize your best life and pinpoint your top priorities and values that you hold dear. What does THE BEST version of your healthy self and life look like?

This includes all elements of your life. Your body, mind and spirit. The environment around you. Your family members. Lifestyle. EVERYTHING! Put these ideas below and then transfer them to a poster board for you to see on a regular basis. This will be your Vision Board.

What brings you joy? Who brings you joy? What do you want to accomplish in your life? Who will be a part of that journey with you? What are your dreams? What do you want to learn? What do you want in your life? Where do you want to travel? You may have forgotten how to dream. Now is your time to reconnect with those dreams again.

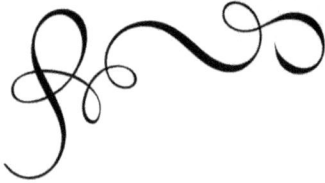

VISION BOARD THOUGHTS

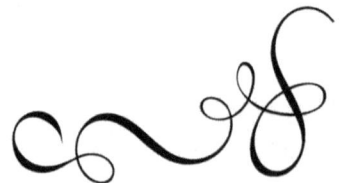

Now, answer this one ... It might feel strange, but this is actually the more important part to dive into as it is more influential on the intended outcome...

What is the worst thing that could happen if you move to a more balanced life, living life on your terms? What/who might get in your way?

If you do not address these and become conscious of them, subconsciously, you will sabotage and allow excuses to run you and you will not gain the life that you so beautifully envisioned above. Please list any reasons that might hold you back if you attain what you want. List any fears and misconstrued beliefs you might have about yourself and your desires. What challenges might you face and who might not like you changing the status quo? What do you not think you deserve? I assure you that these will keep you from attaining your goals if you do not address them thoroughly and honestly. What I have found is that everyone has a 'but', meaning "I would like that in my life, but..." No living in But-land! Now, go! (You may need more room than below.)

WORST THING THOUGHTS

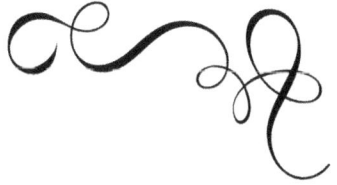

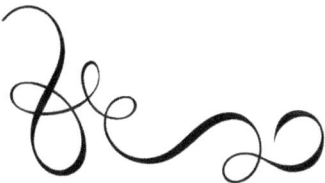

Look at the full vision you want for your life as well as what things might hinder you. Now list out the top priorities/values in your ideal life and put them in order of priority of care. Hopefully, by now you know not to place yourself below anyone else! If there is something you feel is missing, like you forgot to include your kids, or something (oops!), include those elements now. You can also always go back and add! Remember that this is a work in progress and there is no judgment.

Examples might be: God, me, husband, kids, philanthropy, travel, business.

List those here.

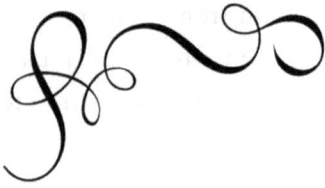 **VALUE LIST**

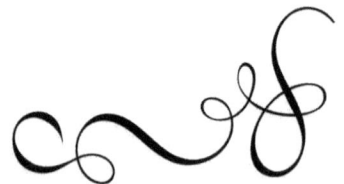

Next, get another large board, or write below and create what I call a "Values Board". This is different from the Vision Board you created above. A Vision Board is your full vision of where you desire your life to be. **A Values Board reflects the main elements on which to concentrate on a daily basis to help you attain that big life vision**. These are your priorities. Once you are finished, display your work somewhere that you will see on a daily basis.

VALUES BOARD THOUGHTS

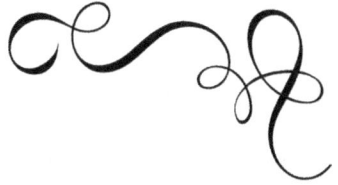

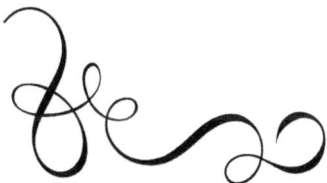

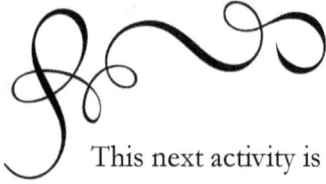

GRATITUDE/GOD PRAYER BOX

This next activity is one of my favorite things to do! If we want to live in a thriving way, no matter the circumstance, we must live in gratitude. If we are breathing, we have something to be grateful for and have a purpose for still being on this planet. Our family has created a Gratitude, or God Prayer Box. This is a box we have in the kitchen where we can write our prayers, or what we are thankful for, on little pieces of paper.

Create one for yourself. This can be something that is out in the open in your home, or something you keep private in your bed stand. Always have pen and paper available and let yourself add to it when you so desire. Let others add to it, if you choose. Pray over your notes and ask God to take care them. Place things in there for which you are grateful, even the most mundane. Living in gratitude can truly change your world, allowing you to be more present and calm in the midst of chaos.

Another example of this is a gratitude wall. In our home we have put up a huge piece of chalkboard fabric covering the wall at the bottom of the stairs with "I am Grateful For…" written big at the top, with a chalkboard marker nearby for anyone to use. It is a blast seeing what our kids write as time goes by, as well as what friends and clients write when they visit. It keeps getting fuller and is a source of happiness in our home. We truly begin to appreciate the smaller, yet beautiful blessings we have in our lives and I invite you to try it.

At the end of this book, you will find a **Gratitude Journal and DONE/ DON'T List** for you to use in the evenings as you work through this book. I invite to you go there on a nightly basis to write at least three things you are grateful for as well as what you accomplished during the day. In doing so, you will increase your confidence, knowing how great your life really is, as well as knowing you accomplished a lot more than you might normally realize. I also invite you to write out your don't's in life.

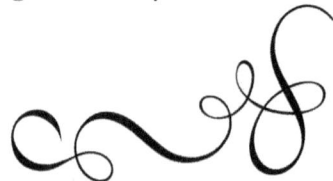

Eli de Moraes

These are things you say "no" to, so that you can say "yes" to better things in your life. We will get more into this later in the book. I hope you enjoy the process as much as I do.

FILL YOUR CALENDAR

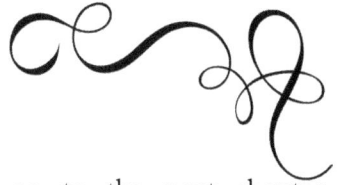

This is a task I ask you to do before you go to the next chapter. Over the coming week, in your calendar, please fill in EVERYTHING you do. This means that when you look at your calendar you will have your normal chunks of time highlighted for appointments, etc., PLUS every single thing you do, including getting up, getting ready, check Facebook, check emails, load dish washer, check Facebook, take kids to school, get lost in Pinterest, get to work, have lunch, get groceries, make dinner, watch TV…you get the picture. It will feel tedious, but it is only for a week and it will give you a good picture needed for an activity we will do later. It is truly imperative for you to write out everything to gain an even more powerful outcome, so push through!

SOLIDIFY YOUR PRIORITIES

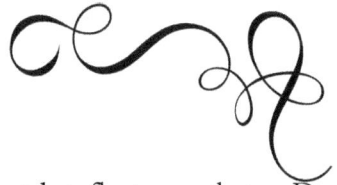

Look at your priorities again. Sit with them and reflect on them. Do they indeed reflect who you are and what you want in life? **Our priorities reflect our values and what drive us.** When we are set with our priorities we are able to create boundaries to protect them from external pressures and tensions in life, thus preventing extra stress from becoming overpowering and debilitating. We can do all the relaxation techniques out there to manage our stress and help us survive, but if we want to truly have a long term, transformational experience, we need to get to the cause of said stress. Nine times out of ten, I assure you that the cause is because somewhere we are not living in tune with our priorities.

So, I invite you now to rededicate yourself to your top priorities. Reflect on your blessings and commit to making everything around you flourish. Ask yourself, what is driving you and get ready to start toning up your life!

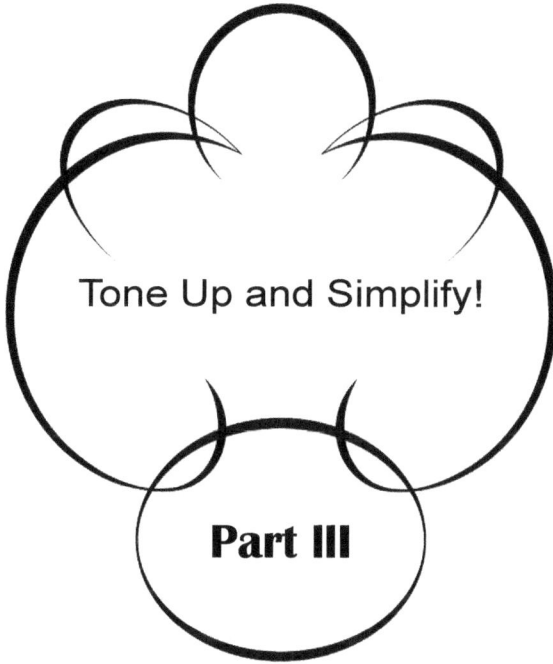

Tone Up and Simplify!

Part III

CHAPTER FOUR

Tone Up Your Life and Simplify, Simplify, Simplify

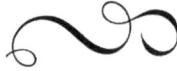

Your next step is to take action in relation to those priorities and simplify by de-cluttering everything in your life! This de-cluttering will include your calendar, activities, home, basic affairs such as doctor appointments, and car and house repairs, as well as your food storage and meal planning. Your goal is to simplify, simplify, simplify, so that life becomes more streamlined, all aspects are organized, and you can go about your life, fully supported with systems in place, without unnecessary stress.

I want you to remember something very important. By letting go of extra 'things' in our lives, whether those are mental, like perfectionism, responsibilities and activities, or actual material things, like 'stuff', negative people, etc., that no longer serve our greater vision of our lives, we make room for better things to come. Do not forget this as you go through everything with a fine-toothed comb.

So, let's first attack that calendar in which you wrote everything!

Take a moment and really sit with your calendar. Take a breath. Take a few deep breaths. Truly look at the reflection of your current life. What does it look like? Does just looking at it give you stress? Now it is time to analyze your activities and see how they align with your priorities and values. We are going to see what can be eliminated as well as what can be delegated. This activity can sincerely be a game changer in your life!

With your Vision and Values Boards nearby, use a color highlighter to highlight EVERYTHING that has nothing to do with your priorities. In a sense, these are your time wasters. This alone will probably free up many hours in the week that you can either get rid of entirely, or consolidate into once-a-day activities such as checking email, Facebook, etc..

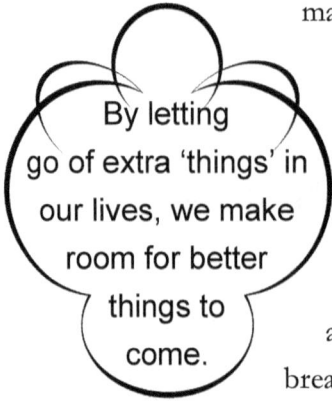

> By letting go of extra 'things' in our lives, we make room for better things to come.

We have to stop the 'pile-it-on' habit. Give yourself permission to time out and let go.

Look also at all the extra activities that you and your family have on the calendar. Do you feel you are running from one thing to another without any breathing room, having to pick up fast food in between? Is everyone completely scheduled out with no down time? If so, it is definitely time to draw the line and pare down those activities. It might seriously pull on you to decrease on this front, as we want to support every interest we and our kids have. However, I assure you that when you do decrease, there will be less stress, anxiety, and yelling and more focused connections made between everyone.

This also goes for all *your* activities, committees and events you are a part of. If you feel constantly rushed and under the gun to get everything finished and there on time, hard truths need to be addressed and dealt with. Something has to go, or keep the concept of dynamic balance in check. If you have a specific timeline of when you can swing back to less chaos with the knowledge that you are choosing to be in this current place that is OK. Otherwise, something has to go. **You cannot be everything to everyone** and lose yourself and your family's state of well-being in the process.

The next step is to take another color highlighter and highlight every single thing that could potentially be delegated, no matter the cost. The reason why I say, no matter the cost, is that I want to you fully look at every aspect of your life where someone else's genius can shine, so that yours can shine where your talents lay, without the blockade that you cannot afford it. At this point in the process, that is irrelevant.

Eli de Moraes

This includes house cleaning, daily household pick up, cooking, grocery shopping, carpooling, laundry, yard maintenance, money budgeting, paper shredding, appointment setting, emptying and loading the dish washer, filing papers, taxes, your online presence if you have a business (web page development, opt-ins, etc.). The list goes on and on.

Now it is time to get into action and attack that calendar and change things around! For the sake of your health and well-being, get rid of anything that does not work toward your greater vision of your life. There are a lot of time wasters that you can put boundaries around. Let them go and stick with it. It feels amazing!

The following are a few examples, but I am sure you will find more.

Can you get rid of your Facebook app on your phone so that you aren't tempted to peek at it? Can you check and respond to emails only once, or twice a day?

Another thing to get rid of is pushing papers through the house. When mail comes in, open it, and respond appropriately and immediately. This means paying the bill on the spot, file it in its proper folder or file it in the recycle bin. If you touch those papers once, and only once, you declutter your house and your time. Don't be a paper pusher from one spot to another.

This next one might be tough, but how about that friend that calls every day and only wants to gossip, or complain about everything? You might need to do some people clearing as well. Create some closure on all aspects that are not positive influences in your life. I assure you that in doing so you won't feel so pulled and won't know what to do with your freer, less stressed time after completing this task! We will address creating more boundaries later in the book.

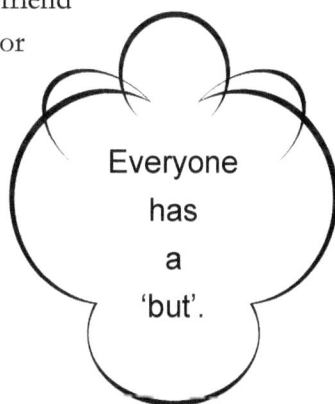

Everyone has a 'but'.

Next, look at what you can delegate. This part is fun! Who else might enjoy, benefit, or learn from doing what you normally do, so to free up some of your time?

What chores can you add to the kids' responsibilities? Can you possibly pay them extra to do something extra? How about hiring an assistant to work a couple of hours on the tasks you find tedious? Wouldn't that allow you to work more on money-making skills if you own a business?

Can you hire someone to come and clean the house every two weeks? I have to tell you that I held out on getting cleaning people for years, but when I finally made the jump it felt like I seriously won the lottery! Try it! It is amazing to have that completely off my plate and I am sure you will, too. Once I made the shift and made it a priority, we didn't feel it in the budget as I thought we would.

What can you trade? Can you trade childcare with other families so that you can have free time for yourself, and/or a date night? Maybe you can partner with a couple of other families in the neighborhood and make extra batches of dinner dishes that you then trade. You cook once and BAM! you have meals for the week!

Let your imagination run and you will be delegating like a pro in no time! Remember that it is for everyone's benefit! Responsibility will be taken on, people will be employed and empowered, and most importantly for you, you will be freeing up time for yourself! It's the ultimate in self-care!

List what you are willing to let go of and what no longer serves you. When things come up you have three choices: take action yourself, let it go and not let it bother you, or delegate it.

THINGS TO LET GO OF

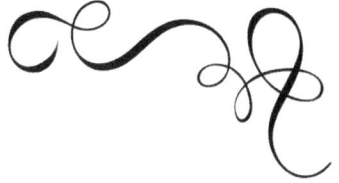

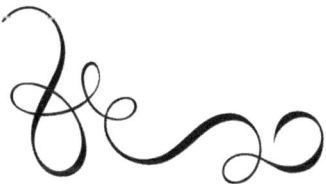

CHAPTER FIVE

Tone up Your Boundaries Around Your Definite Yes's and No's

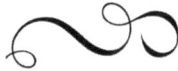

As busy women, often our two greatest challenges are what we say "yes" or "no" to in relationship with how we construct our time. Once we set boundaries around what we allow and not allow in our lives, our schedules tend to become more spacious and malleable. So, let's unapologetically go!

What we say "yes" or "no" to really is about what is important to us. And sometimes what we think is important is not in line with our priorities. If there is discord with how we answer to the pulls in our lives in relation to our values, we gain imbalance in our body, mind and spirit.

For example, your priority might be to lose weight, but you say "yes" to junk food in the house because you don't want it to go to waste. By the action of keeping the food that will tempt you and possibly kick you off your weight-loss journey, you are actually saying that keeping it is more important than losing weight. I am sure that is not the case, unless you desire to sabotage your desired weight loss. By saying "yes" to the stash of junk food, you say "no" to your weight loss. So act on your true values and priorities and donate the food to a worthy cause and focus on the healthy nourishing food your body deserves!

Maybe you have it in your heart to write a book, but you seem to feel that you have to have a clean house before you can start writing each day. You spend your days cleaning up after everyone is out the door, allowing you possibly only an hour to write before it's time to pick up the kids. This, of course, causes anxiety because you aren't following through on your true heart-felt values and what is most important to you. Even if writing that book is everything you have ever wanted to do, your actions show that having a clean house is more important. That is probably not the case, but that is what your actions, or your "yes" to cleaning, says. By saying "yes" to the cleaning, you say "no" to the book. We seem to put self-created parameters around things like having a clean house before we can write that keep us from our goals! Self-sabotage maybe?

So, let's go back to your Values List and highlighted calendar that you wrote earlier. With those in mind, take some time and answer the following.

What are some actions that you have been saying "YES" to that are causing you to say "no" to your values and desires? Write out the statements. For example, "I say 'yes' to a lot of caffeine so that I can keep awake during the afternoon, which means I say 'no' to a good night's rest." Get out a bigger piece of paper for this, if you need.

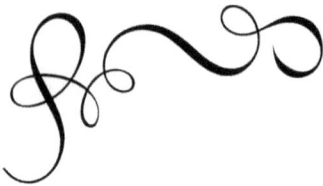

SAY YES TO SAY NO THOUGHTS

It sounds really weird to say these like this, but they are true and hit you right between the eyes when you put them into context like this.

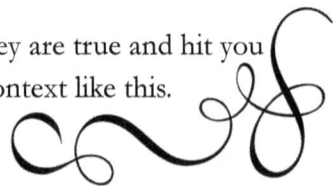

Now do the flip of that. **What are some the actions that you have been saying "NO" to that are making you say "yes" to undesirable things in your life that do not jive with your values and true priorities?** For example, "When I say "no" to taking regular scheduled time for myself, I say "yes" to fatigue and burn out." Again, we are getting honest with ourselves. Go!

SAY NO TO SAY YES THOUGHTS

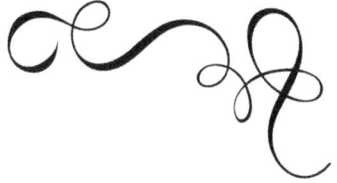

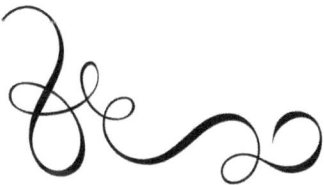

Now, let's flip those and create combined statements that will truly support your values and priorities. For example, "I will say 'no' to TV at night during the week, so that I can say 'yes' to a good night's sleep, which means I also say 'yes' to my desire to have more energy."

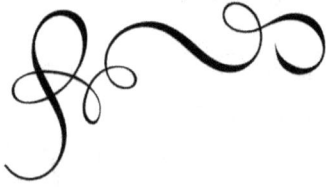

FLIP IT THOUGHTS

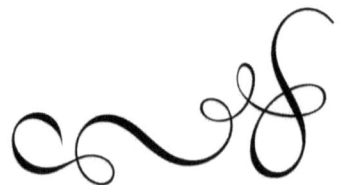

It's pretty powerful stuff, isn't it? Work on catching yourself throughout the day and you will start seeing where your choices can be molded by you, not by your surroundings.

Another way to catch yourself with word usage around your actions that either mis-match, or match your priorities, is to put in "I choose" when you give an explanation with the word 'but' in the sentence. This will cause you to take full responsibility for your actions and remind you that you are the one calling the shots, instead of something external. Of course there are unforeseen circumstances that are completely out of your control, but we are talking about the everyday type of things. When your values are a priority, there are no excuses for you not to follow through on them. If we use the above "yes", "no" and "I choose" statements we really see with what we align.

For example, you might say: "My goal this week was to lose 3 pounds, but because it was so crazy with family in town I over ate and just lost track." In this case, the 'but' gives you an out. Instead say: "My goal this week was to lose 3 pounds, but because it was so crazy with family in town I CHOSE to over eat and just lost track." BAM! WHAAAT? It's the truth, right? This puts the total responsibility back on you. When you see you have choices, you have power.

Or, you might say: "I wanted to go, but I over slept." In this case, you would say, "I wanted to go, but I chose to over sleep." If it was a true priority to get there, you would have set the alarm to get up, but sleeping was more important for you. Of course, mistakes happen, but you get the picture.

With all this in mind, go back to your calendar and integrate some of the "yes" and "no" choices you have been making with time and re-evaluate again.

You want to protect your time and allow your calendar to breathe. **What activities do you still need to cut? What boundaries do you need to set around things like electronics usage, and so forth? Jot down some of your newfound ideas.**

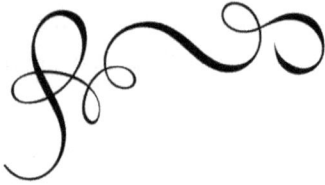

NEW FOUND BOUNDARIES

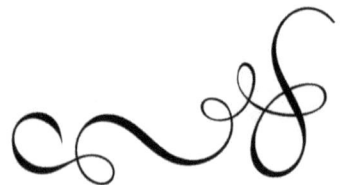

CHAPTER SIX

Tone Up (De-clutter and Define) Your Surroundings

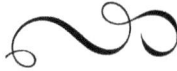

Now get clear on how you want your home to feel and then clear the clutter out of every nook and cranny to support that. This is not for sissies, so get ready to work and let go of things that no longer serve you. Remember that you are opening your space for better things to come, namely peace, energy, happiness and clarity!

Your home needs to be a sacred space for all who live there; a space that represents everyone's values. Be clear on what kind of home you want. Is it a place that is warm and cozy, making people who enter feel loved? It is open and light, making people feel uplifted? Is it bright and colorful to make people feel happy? It is a place that feels peaceful and grounded to recharge all those who enter and live there?

Sit down with your co-habitants and discuss the sense you all want from your home. This will make it easier to get everyone on board. Vision Board-it if you would like.

After you have determined this, do a preliminary sweep through your home and get rid of anything that gives you dissatisfaction, or reminds you of ill things in your life. **If it does not give you pleasure, let it go.** If there is now an empty space, either that is good so leave it that way, or it is now open to be filled with something better when the time is right.

Next, determine the purpose of each room and move things out that do not support that purpose. For example, if it is a bedroom, your work desk (especially!) does not need to be in there.

If it is a guestroom that has become a catch all for all holiday décor, paperwork and out of season clothing, either make a wonderful welcoming place for your guests that is only a bedroom, or put in proper shelving and containers to make it a great and organized place where you can access any of it at a moment's notice. Otherwise, it will remain a black hole that is also not conducive to your guests feeling welcome, or rested. You get the picture. Do this with each room.

Get rid of anything that gives you dissatisfaction.

With the coming step, you will want to create your own plan of attack. And this is where the nitty-gritty work comes into play. We are definitely going to tone your stamina on this one! This is not to scare you, but to prepare you and psych you up! LET'S DO THIS!

It's time to completely declutter EVERYTHING! I like to start on one room at a time, but you might want to take care of all drawers in the house and then all closets, etc. Set a timer for 15-minute increments so that you can play with beating the clock, if you choose, and feel a sense of accomplishment by chinking down your time. Do one 15-minute interval a day, or spend the whole day. It's up to you and what you can afford, time wise. No matter what, do something each day and allow yourself time.

Attack the drawers, closets, cabinets, toy boxes, bookshelves, all paperwork, filing cabinets, and everything else is every room. As you go, see what you want to keep (remember you only keep what gives you joy…you will fill in spaces when the time is right) sell, or give away. Designate their places as you go, so that your space gets clearer and clearer and completely organized. Just think of the clarity you will gain, the money you will make and save, and the joy you will inspire with the articles of which you let go! Save that money either for paying down some debt, so to lessen some stress, or hold on to it so to purchase some things for the home, or your closet, later. Or beef up your savings! Get all family members on board and it will become a fun game and learning experience.

I have found the more simply we live with less clutter, the more satisfied we are with what we have. **I have no idea why, but it seems the more stuff we have the more we want to consume!**

Once you have completed this step you can go on to the next.

Now, as you work through your home, you can always continue onto the other tone-up topics simultaneously, so don't hold yourself back from continuing through the book as you work on the home part. Once you have de-cluttered, it starts getting fun!

Design your home! Create your sacred space that fully expresses who you are.

You have determined what kind of feel you want for the home. You have gotten rid of anything that gives you ill feelings, or what no longer serves you. You are completely organized with everything at your fingertips to create ease. You have designated a certain purpose for each room. Every nook and cranny of your house is decluttered. Now go through and determine furniture placement. Does the traffic flow smoothly? Does each piece serve a specific purpose, either functionally, or aesthetically? Does a piece of furniture block moving through fluidly? Have an outside friend come by and help you with this, as it always helps to have someone that is not so close to it all.

If I am going to get hurt, it is going to happen in bed!

Next, look at lighting for each room in relation to the whole feel you desire in your home environment. Is it too bright? Is it too dim, making it feel gloomy? Does the light bulb have a bluer tone to it, or do you want it to give off a warmer feel? Play with these to set the tone of the purpose of the room. Install inexpensive dimmer switches so that you can change the lighting per your mood. I say this especially for bedrooms and bathrooms so that you can have the ambience you desire, when you desire it. Lighting greatly affects our mood and outlook, so it is important to become clear on this.

Next, start filling in the empty spaces in each room that support your bigger vision for your home as well as the purpose of each room. This step can happen quickly, or as long as you want. I don't suggest that you go out and spend a bunch of money just for the sake of a vision (though that can be super fun!), but do what works best for you.

For example, your bedroom needs calming colors. It needs to feel lush and inviting. Invest in the best mattress and the highest quality sheets that are in your budget. Do not cut corners on either of these as you spend a huge percentage of your entire life here. Remember that you are worth it and need, at the core of your existence, GOOD SLEEP!

I joke that if I am going to get hurt, it is going to happen in bed! Now, get your head out of the gutter! Not THAT way! What I mean is that when I sleep on a mattress that is not good for my body, I can more easily develop chronic back issues, tennis elbow, neck spasms, and more. I say this because you might be suffering from chronic pain and stiffness that are affecting your quality of life. They might simply be taken care of by investing in a better mattress. Supportive pillows are also an option.

Getting back to your bedroom…this room also needs curtains, or shutters that block out all outside light (we will talk about sleep in a later chapter) has soft and adjustable lighting, good airflow, has a nice scent (lavender and cedarwood are great) and NO clutter. If there is clutter, it represents unfinished business, which does not feel good when going to sleep, or when you wake to see it there in the morning.

Over time, go through each room to create the environment you need to support the desires you have for your home. This is your and your family's sacred space. Put as much love and energy into as you wish.

Let me give you an example.

In the process of building our home, in the tilled soil after our groundbreaking, we mixed in glitter (angel dust!...we have two little girls, but I would have done it nonetheless!). Once there was a foundation and a structure, we drew hearts and wrote huge thank you notes to those who were building it on the walls before they were painted.

We invited friends and family to write blessings on the framework around doorways and windows and we also pressed blessed stones in the concrete of the foundation and threshold. We also prayed for and invited God's angels to protect and live amongst us in our home. Love is in all corners and layers here. What I love is that when people come over, they genuinely feel and mention that feeling of peace, love and groundedness built into the very walls and foundation. The intention of the home has been realized.

I say all this to remind you that with each clearing out and addition you make to your home, build love and goodness into it. Your home is your retreat and it, like your body and life, needs to be nourished as such. **You may find that you do this clearing in layers. Allow for this.**

And please know that this all can be done on a shoestring budget all the way through to spending thousands with a decorator who is on the same page as you. You can do this!

Don't forget to continue writing in your Gratitude and DONE/DON'T List Journal!

CHAPTER SEVEN

Tone Up Your General Affairs and Nuisances

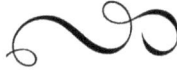

Let's be honest. We often put off what we don't like to do, right? How about those yearly doctor appointments for basic health screenings? Or, how about that mole you have been concerned about? I know some of you might have applied for an extension on your taxes, but are nowhere close to getting them done. And, oops! What about that lost library book you found in the trunk last week?

These are all stressors that only sit and nag at you as you know you need to get them done sooner, or later. I promise when you get all these things cleared out you will feel tons lighter in your step and your mood. So, let's hit it!

List all the things you need to take care of that you have been putting off. Organize them in order of priority and/or deadline. These include things like car repairs, appliance upkeep, finances, record keeping, and doctor's appointments, etc..

GENERAL AFFAIRS LIST

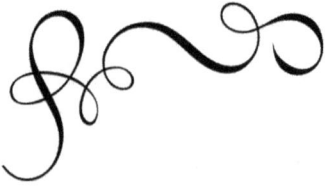

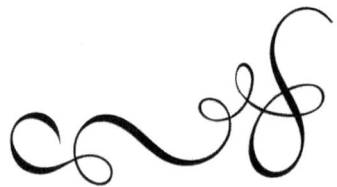

As we continue to flesh through things, let's look at and take care of anything that is a nuisance to you. These are the squeaky doors, the missing cabinet knob, the dead batteries in your house alarm key fob and the loose button on your favorite coat. This can feel tedious, but it will allow you to go through your normal day without those little reminders of what you need to still take care of! Go!

Start your list here and attack them!

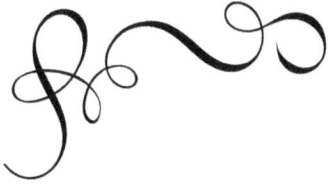

NUISANCES LIST

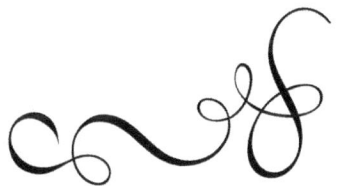

CHAPTER EIGHT

De-clutter and Tone Up Your Food Stash

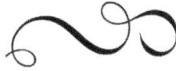

Now for the food part! If you aren't already doing so, as a Health Coach, I am going to invite to reframe your relationship with food to be that of pure nourishment. So often in our hurried state, we develop a relationship with food that is simply something to fill us up when we are hungry. Many of us have unfortunately lost touch with the nourishment, or lack thereof, that food provides. Please, please, please start becoming aware of each bite of food and drink that goes into your mouth and what kind of nourishment and energy it is meant to give you.

My philosophy? Food that is most nourishing is as close to its original LIVING state as possible. The closer it is to its source, the more life it will give our bodies. If it is highly processed, or in a box or bag, I say it is in its coffin as it is dead. If it is dead I know it won't give my body and the bodies I feed in our home the full nourishment they need to thrive. Just think about it.

Now, take EVERYTHING out of your pantry and refrigerator, freezer and deep freeze and put it all on the counter.

Yes, everything.

You might have thought that clearing out your home of everything didn't include these areas, so we have to address them again whether you think you cleaned them out, or not.

THRIVE *Again*

Clean all surfaces of the pantry and fridge to make for a beautiful canvas you are going to create for your food as you put your healthy food back.

Next, dispose of everything that is rotten, or out of date. Yes, that dish you forgot from two weeks ago and those unrecognizable fuzzy 'strawberries' in the back need to go!

Next, you can address your remaining food in two ways:

1. **The money saving mode, but committed to buying healthier food as you go:** If you go this way, you do not care what the nutritional value might be of the food you have bought previously, but don't want to waste anything and want to bring in better food as you go. Put the rest back in the pantry and fridge in an organized manner. If you do this you must be committed to eating up EVERYTHING to clear it out and then only bring in fresh and un-processed food thereafter.

   When my family did this a couple of years ago, it took over a month to eat everything! The recipes were 'interesting' as I was committed to eating up every type of grain, rice and flour we had until it was gone. If I had bought it, it had to be eaten. No longer was I going to let random things just sit in my pantry, or sauces sit in my fridge, for years anymore. Come on! You know you have got to have that old jar of pickles from the Forth of July, 2012, or that Crisco your mom used to bake a pie who knows when! They have to go if you don't know how old they are!

   While we did this plan, I only bought essentials, like milk, eggs, fruits and veggies, but other than that I was determined!

   I have had clients who took months before they ate up everything! By doing so, they reduced waste and saved A LOT of money by not forgetting what they had! The same will happen for you, too.

2. This next method is my preferred one as it puts you on the fast track toward healthier eating. **Here, you are done with processed food, once and for all, and are willing to donate what you can so to have a clean slate as well as bless your local food pantry.**

After you have taken everything out of your food stores, only put back fresh and dry food. Veggies, fruit, grains, meats, etc.

My favorite part? I like to organize and artfully display everything so that our family can honor and enjoy the beauty of the nutrient-rich food that will be nourishing us. I know, I am a complete geek, but I love it! It works! It gets you back to the source and a reminder to care about the nutrients that will allow your body to thrive!

Displaying your non-refrigerated foods on the counter is also a wonderful way to honor your food as you pass by. When you do all this, food no longer becomes just something to fill you when you are hungry, but something that you choose to have to fully nourish you.

We will look at food purchasing in a bit.

FOOD STASH NOTES

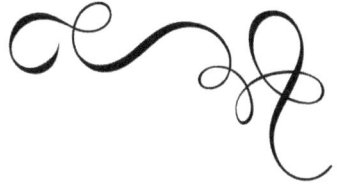

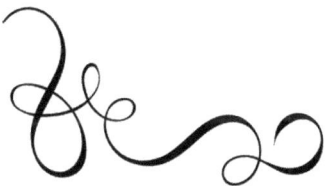

CHAPTER NINE

Feed Your Amazing Body

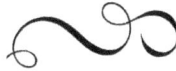

One cannot think well, love well, sleep well, if one has not dined well.
~Virginia Woolf

I love this quote because it is so true in all respects concerning what we 'dine' on and what nourishes all aspects of ourselves. This not only includes the food we put in our bodies, but our relationships, spiritual practices, our home life and so much more! So how are you feeding your body and life?

Our existence depends on our consumption of good food, water, light, sound and love. See each of these as nutrients. You were created to be close to the source: food, community, nature, your body/yourself. It's time to get back to that concept for good reason: your body. It is the vessel that holds your life, the miracle in which you experience life, and the creative vessel that generates life.

Let me first give you some statistics from one of my mentors, Dr. Libby Weaver at the Institute of Integrative Nutrition. When you understand how utterly amazing your body is, you will start to walk around a bit taller, due to knowing what kind of miracle you are! You will probably also be more motivated to feed it well on all fronts. Can you believe that we have trillions of cells in our bodies? Trillions!

The outer layer of our skin renews itself every month and we are blessed by a replaced blood supply every three months!

Can you believe that on average our heart:
- beats 100,000 times per day
- pumps 2000 gallons of blood through
- 60,000 miles of blood vessels in just one body?!? Crazy!

As adults, we create a new skeleton every 10 years and children do it every year!

I am a TOTAL geek when it comes to learning about the body as it is a complete miracle. We experience everything through our own, unique body. **Take a moment to ponder this.**

Sit and breathe. Feel that precious air enter your nostrils and fill your lungs. Rub your hands together and feel the touch, the warmth and friction. Look around. Really SEE your surroundings. Now stand up and start stretching and moving your body in all directions, 3-dimensionally.

Now, just walk across the room. Consider all the nerves, tendons, ligaments and muscles involved in that simple act and the specific order in which they had to function to make it a smooth operation! And all that happened with virtually no conscious thought at all! You certainly weren't thinking about which muscles needed to move. Isn't it all amazing?!? The body truly puts me in awe!

Always remember that never in the history of all humankind has the collection of cells come together to make up a person just like you. And because of that, there is absolutely no telling what you can accomplish in your lifetime. Do not let anyone (especially yourself) tell you that you have to be a certain way and that you can only accomplish certain things. I tell you this so that you might become even more motivated to nurture and nourish your body and life. You want to keep those cells functioning at their optimal levels for as long as they can, so together they act as a vessel for you to experience the most out of your life as possible!

If we want to ensure proper functioning and rejuvenation as well as avoid developing chronic diseases, we must supply the body with the right nutrients. So, let's address your food, movement, and mindset.

CHAPTER TEN

Tone Up Your Meal Planning

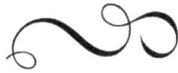

One of my biggest challenges in running our household is meal planning. I am the first to admit that I am the queen of, "Oh, it's 5pm and have no idea what we are having for dinner!" I have never been good at it and would downright avoid it, if it wasn't so freaking amazing for decreasing my stress levels when I *do* plan! Because I have had such issues with it, I have searched out ways to help, so let me outline different levels one can take. Use one, or combine a few to create something that works for you.

1. **Meals-by-Improv method.** This is what I spoke about that I am prone to do, but for our family, this lack of pre-planning does not warrant a very good outcome. I get stressed, feel guilty that I am not a good mom for not thinking about it, and end up making less healthy choices due to people becoming 'hangry'. This causes more guilt.

   Now, others thrive on this type of planning, if you can call it that. They can easily look in the fridge and pantry and whip up a divine concoction fit for a 5-star restaurant! If this is how you roll, I bow down to you! Continue on!

2. **Calendar planning.** This is done by sitting down once a week to plan out the week's food. You simply pick out your favorite recipes for each meal, put them in your calendar and plan out what you need to put on

your shopping list for your ONCE A WEEK grocery shopping. If you desire, you can repeat the same the following week, so to save yourself the hassle of planning again, but your family may not be keen on that.

If this is too intensive, you can use various online services to aid you in such. At the time of publication of this book, I have various resources you can access. A couple of sources are:

Buying seasonally will create diversity in your choices.

www.PlanToEat.com. This is one of my favorite ways to plan our week! It utilizes calendar planning, but on a whole new level by taking out a lot of the grunt work of searching all over for recipes, writing out grocery lists and more.

You can go into their large database of recipes (or add more from other sources), pick out which ones you desire and put them in your own account. From there, you can then click on which recipes you want and drag them into your desired meal spot on the provided calendar! Once you do this, it populates your shopping list for you! Genius!

There are also other online tools, such as www.thescramble.com, that will send you your menus along with shopping lists.

There are many out there, so search for what works best for you and your budget.

Big cooking tips for when you plan as above:

• Cook multiple batches to freeze. You cook once and eat multiple times. Cook for one week, eat for two!

• You can also partner up with other families and trade those extra batches and voila! You have yourself diverse meals for the week!

• Repeat your weekly plans two times in a row, or create four weeks of meals and repeat monthly. This saves you time and allows you the ability to not have to be too creative all the time.

- I like to designate one day a week (it's Sunday in this household) for cooking for the week. I literally take everything out of the refrigerator to see what we have. This gives me a chance to repurpose any left-overs, see what ingredients I can use for the coming week and clean up the ridge. This one action has saved us from forgetting, and as a result, throwing out food. When we designate one day we also cook once and clean ONCE! Plus, all I have to do is pull a meal out when needed during the week because it has been prepared in advance. When I do this type of cooking, I do not designate certain menus for certain days as I like to see what our mood is on a certain day. All I have to know is that there are enough meals in the fridge or freezer for the week and I am good.

Cooking this way also allows me to know what ingredients I might be missing so that I can go one time to the store. This avoids wasting any time going multiple times in a week to shop.

I also enjoy prepping it all on a day where everyone is at home so that it becomes a family affair.

- Some people like to cook and freeze for the whole month. I have never gotten myself motivated to do this, but I think it rocks if you can do it! Just think…no cooking for a month! Brilliant! But you need a biiiig freezer.

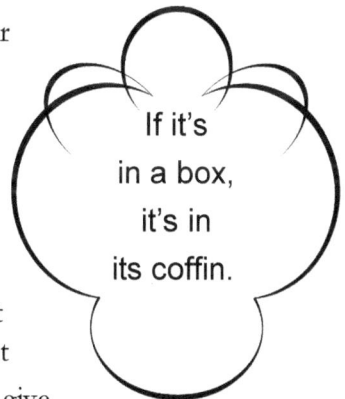

If it's in a box, it's in its coffin.

- Something special I like to do to connect myself with the food, is to take a moment before I begin prepping it, to be silent, give honor to the food that will nourish us, and pray over it to bless us. This one act shifts the chore of cooking to one that feeds my soul. Try it!

3. **The next level of planning is utilizing one of the online, home delivery meal companies** like Hello Fresh, Plated, Blue Apron and many more. Each week, these companies send you the necessary pre-portioned ingredients for each meal they have planned. You determine how many meals you want each week, for how many people for whom you want to cook. These can be on the pricier side, but are great for those of us who do not want to have to plan anything, or who want to be exposed to new cooking ideas. Each company out there has a different focus for different people's needs. Some are all organic. Some are geared for the Paleo diet. Search around and you are bound to find what works for your dietary needs.

4. **The next level of planning is to have a personal chef plan out and cook your meals.** This is, of course, more expensive than the other ways of planning. But if you are a busy high-level business woman with intense work demands, and can afford it, this will allow you more time to focus on your priorities, like your family and your down time. This level may seem extreme, but I invite you to see it as a gift of an ultimate tool in self-care. If you can afford it and cooking is not one of your favorite things to do, hire your personal chef today! You will feel like you won the lottery! That's one more thing on your to-delegate list checked off! I have never had one, but boy, when my business is making 6-figures +, I certainly look forward to taking that off my plate!

CHAPTER ELEVEN
Tone Up Your Food Shopping

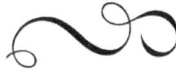

If you haven't already figured out, I want you to cook the majority of your meals, at home, with REAL and fresh food that is in season. We often lose touch with our roots, bodies, and nature while eating fast 'franken-', or processed food that just fills us up, and makes us sick in the long run. When we cook in the home with fresh food, we get closer to our source and are empowered to health.

"But where should I buy those ingredients, Eli?" you might ask! I would love to answer that!

My first choice is always going to be your local farmers market. When you shop these establishments, you support and get to know your local farmers who grow and nurture your food. You can more easily find out how they really grow their crops and you can make informed decisions from there.

A cool thing to know about farmers markets is that if you are looking to buy organic you will often be able to get it less expensively than at the grocery store. If something is sold as 'organic' at the store, the farmer has to pay high fees to label it as such. At the market, you may find someone who sincerely grows organically, but does not jump through all the hoops, or incur huge expenses to get the official labeling. This means they do not pass those expenses onto you! Because you have hopefully developed a relationship with them, you can more readily believe that they are telling the truth. Of course, this is per your judgment, but I know at our market, each farmer must undergo extensive vetting and impromptu tours of their farm to be approved to sell there. I also trust my intuition, but to each his/her own.

You also help the environment by supporting farmers who drive their crops usually only within a 100-150 mile radius, rather than 100s, if not, 1000s of miles to get to you at the store. It is a small, yet large gesture all around when you shop your farmer's market.

One of my favorite aspects of a market is that you are forced to buy and eat seasonal food for your specific region. This is because that is all that can grow there. Our bodies are meant to eat various foods throughout the year and this is accomplished when we eat closer to the land.

People wonder why they develop allergies to certain foods all of a sudden when they have always eaten them. That's your answer. You may develop sensitivities if you only eat a certain selection of foods for breakfast, lunch and dinner that you get at the grocery store. These are usually foods from all over the world that are not intended for your region to eat all the time. I am not saying not to eat international food. How would I be able to drink my coffee or favorite wine, or eat my favorite international fare? What I am saying is that we are not meant to have bananas on our oatmeal with orange juice every single morning, every single day of the year. Buying seasonally will create diversity in your choices, allowing your body to be nourished with variation.

Your next shopping choice is, of course, the grocery store. The biggest recommendation I have for you here is to focus primarily on the outer perimeter of the store. This is where all the fresh food is kept, allowing you to stay with healthier choices and not be tempted by processed goodies and not-so-truthful marketing and packaging.

Do NOT be tempted by packaging that says 'natural', 'fortified', or any other misdirection. First of all, 'natural' labeling nowadays is often so far from true and, second, if it says 'fortified' that only means that they have processed it so much, that it is now lacking nutrients and need to add back in nutrients that are not as bio-available, or accessible for our bodies to absorb. Just don't go there. As I mentioned earlier, my philosophy is that if it is in a box, or bag, it is dead and in its coffin. If is it processed, it is too far from its original living state and not fully fit to nourish your body. This type of food only causes more strain on the body systems and right now, we are all about decreasing the stress load, right? I am not saying to feel bad when you buy processed food. Just be aware and decrease the amount that you buy.

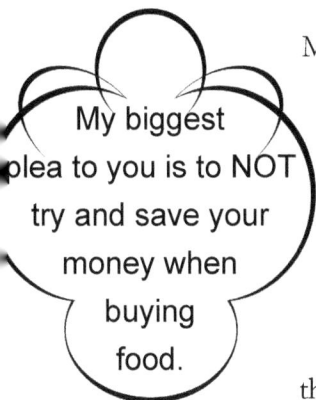

> My biggest plea to you is to NOT try and save your money when buying food.

My biggest plea to you is to not try and save your money when buying food. Yes, shop sales on your fresh foods, but please work to save your money on other things. I am sure that if you put your food and your health on top priority you will find that other extraneous things are not so high on the list. You might save on food now, but I assure you that you are more likely to have higher medical bills later, plus everything else that comes from illness, if you do. This mindset away from coupon clipping (which, by the way, usually motivates you to buy more boxed, franken-food, right?) can take a bit, but I am sure you can cut corners on other things.

Simply taking out fast-food treks will save you a ton of money, so invest in nourishing food, starting today.

I will say that since I switched our home to primarily fresh food that is bought once a week, rather than having large amounts stored in a full pantry and freezer, we spend less money on food. We waste less and are more connected to what we are eating. We also don't forget what food is in our house and don't get sick as often.

I have to share a little funny thing with you. We recently had a sleepover party for our 12 year old daughter. In the evening when the girls were looking for some snacks to eat, they asked if they could look through the pantry. To their surprise there wasn't anything in there except ingredients! Nothing, except for a little stash of candy my girls have, was pre-made, or boxed! They made fresh air-popped popcorn and cut up a bunch of fruit and veggies and were happy as clams. This goes to show you that you don't have to have a bunch of junk to make kids happy. If they are hungry, they will eat what you put in front of them. If they don't eat it, they will not go hungry, I promise you. Primarily have good food on hand and you will take care of many potential health and behavioral issues.

So, if getting your family on board with eating differently is a concern for you, rest assured that they will end up thanking you for the change, no matter the initial difficulty. They will have more energy, you all will probably weigh a healthier weight and feel the nourishment you all need. Patience.

Write in any thoughts you might have and don't forget your Gratitude Journal!

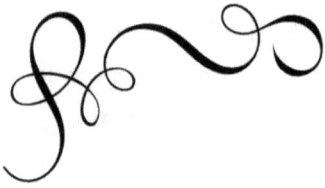

THOUGHTS ON FOOD SHOPPING

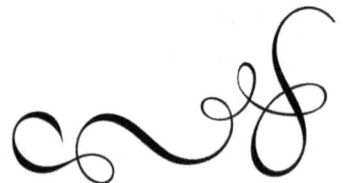

CHAPTER TWELVE

Understand Your Eating Patterns and Why We Hold On To Weight

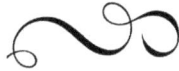

In this section I invite you to look at your eating patterns and your relationship with food. Do you eat dependent on your mood, or when you are authentically hungry? Do you eat because you are bored, or lonely?

Food literally fills us up, physically and mentally, so if we are to have a healthy body, we have to be honest with ourselves and confront the hard facts and make changes where needed.

If you happen to be overweight, I need you to let go of one big elephant that I know is probably in the room. YOU ARE NOT FAT BECAUSE YOU LACK WILLPOWER, or are lazy! You are overweight because of the types of food you have eaten that have caused imbalances in your body so that you cannot access the fat to lose it. When we get into certain cycles, those foods and those imbalances cause us to crave and physically need to eat certain things that are less healthy. In saying this, our fat literally makes us fatter!

Now, I cannot determine your specific causes without working with you in person, but I bet you have developed a number of things, like insulin resistance, that are making it more difficult to shed the weight.

My recommendation is to find a good practitioner who will help you uncover some of the challenges that are happening in your body and address them with the right foods, but also look at the reasons you are where you currently are. In saying this, make sure this person's philosophy of weight loss is not a one-size-fits-all regimen. You will also want to look at what fears you might have if you do lose weight, just like we looked at when creating the Vision Board.

Let's look at some of the psychological aspects of weight.

Looking at your fears may sounds strange, but I assure you that if you do not address them, you will either sabotage yourself every step of the way with excuses, or gain it all back in the coming months when you are confronted by whatever you might be afraid of. This is one reason why so many people are able to lose weight with hard core calorie restriction and high intensity exercise, but then only gain it all back in six months, causing a never ending cycle of weight fluctuation and poor self-esteem.

One fear I hear come up is that you might be afraid of the new attention you might gain from potential partners if you lose the weight. It is so interesting how, in our society, you can become more invisible, the bigger you are. If we are afraid of the attention, we might allow ourselves to get bigger. We might also use our weight as an excuse, or a way to sabotage ourselves so to not fully reach for our goals for fear of not attaining them. We might use our weight as a reason in our minds why we might not fully get there, rather than our potential lack of talent, or skill. I know I did this during my time as a professional dancer.

> Many times we confuse dehydration with hunger.

There I was, dancing all over the world, but my weight would fluctuate, depending on my level of confidence in myself and in relation to my fears. If I thought I was getting too close in having to trust in myself, I got bigger. I felt amazing when I was dancing, but was convinced my weight would hold me back. If my weight held me back, I would never have to know if it was really my lack of talent that kept me from succeeding.

If I didn't know that talent threshold because my weight was there, I could always blame the weight, rather than my potential lack of talent. It sounds crazy, but that was what I was working with. When the director of the Helsinki (Finland) Ballet told me that I didn't deserve to be on stage due to my weight, this belief was proven. We will leave fate to determine his destiny for saying such a disgusting thing, but I fulfilled my prophecy. My weight stopped me at a certain level and I didn't have to know where my true talent threshold was.

I also found that, on the flipside, I was afraid of my power. I was afraid of how far I could really go, and at that time I couldn't wrap my head around it, or accept that I was worthy of it. I could feel the power inside of me that I knew was of God, but I was afraid of it. Yes, again, that sounds crazy, but I am being honest. I still struggle with this, as I know many of us do, but I am getting better. I believe the majority of us are probably afraid of our God-given power, thus live more stressful lives fighting it.

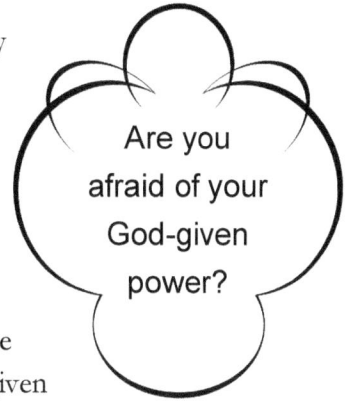

Are you afraid of your God-given power?

On another note, I was also dealing with a silent emptiness that I thought could only to be filled with food. I could go out with friends for dinner and come home alone and eat an entire box of cereal. I was never bulimic, but I was definitely addicted to food and could secretly pack it away. Of course this really wasn't a secret because the extra pounds on my body gave me away. This, also, did not help parts of my dance career as my weight fluctuated while on the road on tour.

I tried all sorts of tricks to help me lose weight, from extreme diets and full body ice baths to rev up my metabolism, to body wraps. None of those things worked for long as I wasn't really addressing the real issues as to why I had gotten more than 30 pounds heavier than I am today.

I have to tell you that the moment that emptiness in me got filled, the weight literally fell off in a rather short amount of time. And I haven't had a weight issue since because my relationship with food changed. Also, I started eating food that nourished me, rather than fought me, and now my body has found a happy medium. I listen to what it needs at each stage of my life and change accordingly.

Every once and a while I can indulge in what is considered junky, but because I am no longer addicted to food and my body's metabolism is functioning at a more optimal rate, I can afford to 'cheat' here and there without guilt. Because certain things got filled in my life, the addiction went away. I also now know how to rein myself in to a healthier way of eating. Other parts of my me got fed and the weight became a non-issue.

This is why weight loss is not a simple one-size-fits-all restricted calorie, heavy-duty workout, type of thing that so often is touted as THE way to lose weight in our society. First of all, it is not always the amount of calories you eat. It is the TYPE of calories you consume. One has to also look at all sides of one's life such as relationships, career, fears, and so much more. You are unique with a certain heritage, genetic make-up, sensitivities, a certain lifestyle and a life story that is literally embodied in every cell of your body.

To live a thriving healthy life, you want to find what types of foods work best for your specific body and lifestyle. And please know that what is perfect for my body might be poison for yours.

Find the type of foods that work best for your specific body and lifestyle.

I have a client who is a vegetarian. She is lean and looks absolutely amazing. When looking at the big picture, one might think that her way of eating is THE way to lose weight and look great because it works for her. My answer is no, not for everyone. If I eat like her, I get puffy, bloated and gain weight. I know my body needs animal protein at my age and stage in my life to function optimally. The same might be for you.

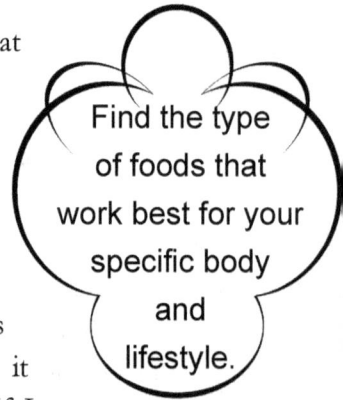

What this means, again, then, that certain popular diet plans may not be for you. You might try them without success and feel like you failed. In reality they failed you because they were not the right fit for you. So, that being said, a gluten-free, Paleo, vegetarian, or high carb diet may not be the answer for you. Find someone who can help you navigate this discovery process for your specific body so that you can find what works for you and supports your system in the best way possible. When you do this you will be golden!

Other simple tips concerning weight gain and weight loss:

- Don't drink your calories. Be aware of what you are drinking because extra calories by way of sugars get hidden in many drinks out there. If you drink sodas, juices and specialty coffees, you will be amazed at how quickly some of your extra weight will slide off by simply adding more water instead. In doing so, you will often automatically start decreasing those types of drinks. This goes for diet drinks as well. Studies show that the artificial sweeteners in diet drinks and treats can cause you to feel hungrier, thus causing you to eat more. Remember what I said about being aware of the types of calories, not so much the amount?

- My rule: water is what your body craves, so drink it as your main source of hydration. **Many times we confuse dehydration with hunger** and end up eating more, so grab a glass before anything. I have a glass by my bedside to drink first thing each morning to rehydrate my body after no extra water during the night. This not only curbs hunger, but it also helps to hydrate the brain, which will help you have a clearer mind. And, of course, the rest of the body gets hydrated to work with less struggle and stress.

- The same type of thing happens when we lack sleep. Women in particular, confuse sleepiness with hunger and then go for what feels like a quick energy booster by medicating with sugar and/or carbs. Instead, drink a glass of water first, and work toward getting adequate sleep. Getting fuller rest will help decrease your cortisol levels, which can help you lose weight. The sleep discussion is coming in a bit!

- When you have a craving to eat, fill it by addressing its source. Are you truly hungry? If so, figure out exactly what your body needs and fill it. If you are not hungry, but reaching for food due to boredom, anxiety, or loneliness, do something else that will satisfy that craving, or emptiness. Go for a walk, call a friend, or meditate, for example.

- Get your blood work done. You might have certain nutrient deficiencies that if you get those taken care of, you might fix many issues. The same might be for your hormones.

- Play with different types of food and see what works for you and what doesn't. Doing so, will help you understand what they do to you and what you should avoid. An elimination diet can truly help you with this. If you have brain fog, inflammation and unexplained weight gain, this might help you get the bottom of it.

- Remember that the more stress we have, the less our bodies can assimilate the nutrients we give it, which can aid in holding onto weight. When we stay in the 'fight or flight' state we also are not as readily able to access the fat in our body. Chill out and lose weight, my friends!

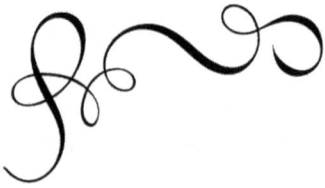

THOUGHTS ON YOUR EATING PATTERNS

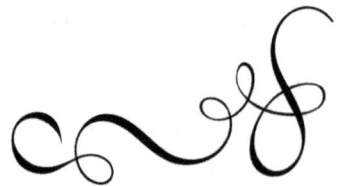

CHAPTER THIRTEEN

Tone Up Your Body Through Finding Joy in Moving

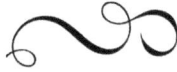

As certain foods work better for your body's make-up, the same goes for your exercise and movement. Dependent upon your body type, nervous system and personality, you will find what works best for you. Go out and experiment. Find what you have fun doing and what feels good in your body. For me, that is dancing. When I dance, I feel alive, fully in my body and invincible. For you, that might mean walking in nature, surfing, planting a garden, wakeboarding, kick boxing, or doing yoga. Find that sweet spot and keep doing it because a big key to you living a thriving life to is to just keep moving.

The longest living humans on our planet do not have gym memberships. They have gardens. They walk. They commune with nature. They dance in celebrations. They have a purpose in life and live it. They LIVE.

I can write an entire other book on exercise and movement, but my main intention here is to help you grasp the concept that the best thing to do for yourself is to find something that gives you joy through moving. As a yoga and Pilates teacher, I could easily tell you that those forms are THE best for you. Although I fully believe in the transformational qualities that those modalities provide, I know that every form of exercise has its benefits. It is your job to find what works for you.

I do want to give one word of caution. Often what we are naturally attracted to is what will put us off balance. For example, you might be a type A personality who is a go-getter CEO of a company. You might be more drawn to a high intensity hot yoga, or a boot-camp-style class because you feel you need to burn off some steam. Unfortunately, those can actually fuel the fire that is inside you even more and cause you to go into overdrive and overextend an already exhausted nervous system.

You might say that a traditional, non-hot, yoga class is too slow and boring for your fast-paced mind and body. In actuality, a slower, more sustained form of body work is exactly what you need to balance you. You will calm the sympathetic nervous system out of the fight or 'flight mode', which will allow you to get stronger, yet calmer through your parasympathetic system. The opposite is true if you are more prone to moving slowly. You may need a little kick in the butt to rev things up! Remember that too much of anything will take you off balance, so choose wisely and be in tune with what you really need and enjoy.

Our bodies are meant to move, so have at it! It will also help reduce stress and release endorphins that can make you stronger and feel more alive and energetic. The more you enjoy the type of exercise you do, the more you will do it. There is a beauty in movement. Cultivate it!

CHAPTER FOURTEEN

Breathing Does a Body Good

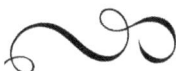

Breathing is the most fundamental element of living. We can go without food and water for weeks, without the heart beating for minutes, but without air, we will die very quickly. It is what gives us our life energy.

In our hurried 'fight or flight' lives we can easily find ourselves primarily breathing shallowly and high in the chest. We feel like we are dragging our bodies along like heavy ragdolls full of fatigue. We do not know how to break the cycle. Because we forget to breathe deeply, this causes us to have a lack of oxygen to feed our brains and bodies.

In response, let's **take a moment to connect with our breath and be still.**

As you read this, sit up tall so to literally give your lungs and organs space to breathe. Now gift yourself four deep breaths from the bottom of your lungs. Let your belly expand. Close your eyes and repeat.

Feel your body fill up with all the sweetness in your life. Think of breathing life into your life. There are countless blessings, so breathe them in.

Let's go back to that memory of a great smell from food. Think about that time when you entered your home, or the home of a loved one, where someone had baked, or cooked your favorite dish. The memory of that fragrance brings such joy and love into your being. Remember those feelings and let them permeate every cell of your body.

How do you now feel? Tingly? Alive? Joyful? All of the above? It's amazing what the simple act of deep breathing can do for our body, mind and spirit. Whenever stressed, or actually as often as you can think of it, do this exercise. I know there are many simple things that can rock your world and this is one of them!

To counter that 'fight or flight' mechanism, and that shallow, stress-inducing breathing mentioned above, we want to activate the parasympathetic nervous system with diaphragmatic breathing. Have you ever watched a baby, or someone sleeping, and noticed their belly rising and falling? This is diaphragmatic breathing. It helps to cultivate the 'rest and digest' mechanism, allowing us to breathe more fully and to chill out. It is what you just practiced if you truly breathed deeply. You can access this form of breathing any time and I recommend putting a timer on throughout the day to remind yourself to do it.

Another breathing practice is alternate nostril breathing. You can use your thumb and ring finger to block off each alternate nostril as you practice, but you can also just imagine it. This form of breathing helps to calm and balance your body and mind. You can use it while driving, while in the boardroom, or while trying to fall asleep when the mind is stressed, or racing. And what is cool is that no one needs to be the wiser and know what you are doing. Instead of Valium, or Ambien, just do alternate nostril breathing!

To begin, visualize inhaling through the right nostril and out the left. Inhale through the left and out the right. This is one cycle. Repeat as long as you desire.

If trying to get to sleep, lie on your right side and do 8 cycles. Then, do 16 cycles on your left side. Next, get on your back and do 32 cycles. To be honest, I never make it to my back! Try it out.

Another breathing concept that I love to use is playing with the length of exhale in relation to the inhale. The longer the inhale, the more energy you will gain and the longer the exhale the more relaxed energy you will develop.

For example, when you have that mid-day slump where your first instinct is to grab a coffee, I invite you to sit up tall and start this newly learned breathing technique. Determine a count that works for you. You might inhale for 6 counts and exhale for 3, or 4. Continue for a bit and you will feel the difference. This is also good for those long road trips where the monotony of the road can take its toll. Instead of grabbing another cup of coffee, practice your breathing. Now, if you are super sleepy, listen to your body and get off the road for some sleep. There is no reason to push the body to extremes and put yourself and others at risk. If your body needs rest, your ultimate priority is to give it what it needs.

The reverse is true if you are anxious, had a run-in with someone, just about had it with the kids, or simply want to calm the mind to get to sleep. Flip the numbers and count to 3 or 4 on your inhale and 6 for the exhale. You will soon feel a sense of calm and peace with a calmer mind.

Breathing can be your constant companion that helps to regulate the body. Breathing and the body are intricately intertwined and if the breathing is off, the body is off. And if the body is off, the breathing will also usually be off. Start by focusing the breath and the body will follow.

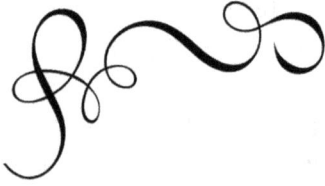

BREATHING THOUGHTS

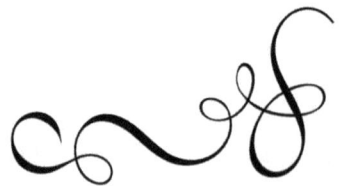

CHAPTER FIFTEEN

Mindfulness and Meditation Make a Difference

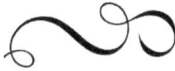

In our rushed lives, we can mentally be in multiple places by planning a meeting later in the day, remembering we need to rush to the grocery store between the kids' flute and Taekwondo lessons, texting your best friend about the PTO meeting you're leading tomorrow, calling the school to inform them that Sally will not be in school today because you found lice on her head, and emailing the city about a water leak you noticed on the corner of your street. Whew! That stresses me out just reading it.

Through all this we need to learn to embrace the beauty of the chaos when it comes. Through mindfulness we allow ourselves to relish and savor the sweetness of a simple single sensation, or occurrence within the cacophony of the mind's chatter. It helps us to break rhythms, and honor and see the beauty in the mundane so to let go of the chokehold we can have on everything else.

I invite you to find sweet spots throughout the chaos of your day. Find those "pinch-me, is this real?" moments of grace and beauty. It takes practice, but you can find those moments more readily through practicing meditation.

Meditation helps develop a single-pointed concentration, helps calm the mind, slows your reactions, helps you become healthier, and aids you to be more joyful and at peace and in the present.

THRIVEAgain

So to ease you into this practice I offer you a few simple meditations. Start with short periods of time, like 2 minutes, and work to grow from there. It takes time to develop that mediation muscle to stay single-focused without the mind wandering. If you find that the mind does wander, simply witness the thoughts, let them go and refocus on the single task at hand.

Simple Medtations:

- While walking, feel your feet on the ground

- Simply sit still and listen to the sounds around you

- Go out in nature to attune your body, mind, spirit and breath to the rhythms of life. This means to listen and feel the surroundings

- Be mindful of every breath

- Watch the clouds go by, or watch the grass grow.

- Simply do the breathing techniques described previously.

- Sit and stare into a candle. Watch the flame and simply focus on it.

Another support in learning to be more present in the moment as well as help your body access the parasympathetic nervous system is deep relaxation.

Additional benefits of deep relaxation include increased immunity, emotional balance and a lowering of blood pressure. It is calming, anti-inflammatory, and you might lose weight. It also helps to decrease cortisol plus supports the adrenals, which then strengthens your immune system. You get sick less and heal faster. It might also help you live more with a sense of gratitude, supporting you through the chaos.

Some techniques include: guided relaxation, Yoga Nidra (further described in a bit) and restorative yoga. I recommend searching online, or find a local yoga teacher to teach you these in person.

Please write any thoughts you might have on the following pages and do not forget your Gratitude Journal writing in the back!

THOUGHTS ON MINDFULLNESS/MEDITATION

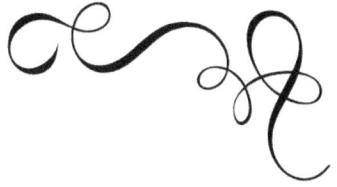

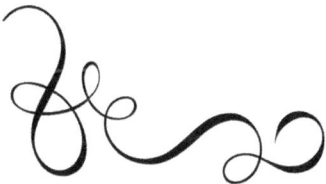

CHAPTER SIXTEEN

Tone Up and Recommit to Good Relaxation & Sleep

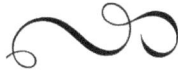

Take a rest; a field that has rested gives a bountiful crop. ~Ovid

Caution! Good sleep can cause: weight loss, better concentration, less cravings for sugar and carbs, better problem solving, creativity, alertness, less discomfort, and a stronger immune system causing you to be less likely to develop chronic illnesses and auto-immune disorders.

Those who are sleep deprived often get more easily irritated, have poor digestion, have more accidents, are less productive, are more prone to multi-tasking (and you know the rule on multi-tasking!), and of course, are more prone to illness

We all need more rest, but please do not confuse rest with recreation and/or inebriation. Those can add to what we think is rest, but we all need more SLEEP! Begin to think of sleep as something sacred and vital for your optimal vitality. Sleep is not 'not awake' or something we just have to go and do because we are tired.

Please list what you hope good sleep will do for you, personally.

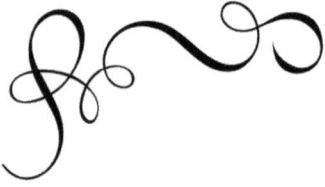

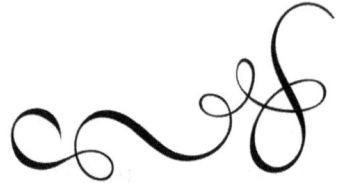

List reasons why you presently don't get good restful sleep (if you don't).

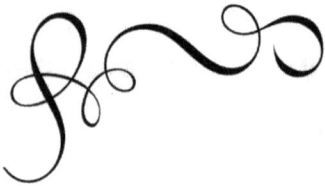

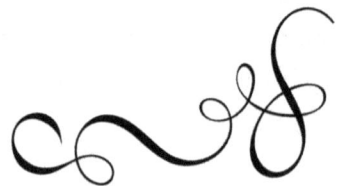

When we get good sleep, so many other health issues become obsolete, so I invite you take this very seriously.

There are many factors that affect sleep, but one big cause that is easily rectified is ones evening ritual of settling down for the night. Until modern history, we went to bed when the sun went down. Once it starts getting dark we start producing melatonin, but because of electricity and the blue light that is emitted from the screens of our computers, phones and TVs, our body gets confused that it is still daytime and does not naturally create the hormones it needs for deep sleep. Try to keep electronics off at night at all costs. I know it is hard, but worth the benefits of sleep.

Also, think about the activities you have in the evening. If you have to rev up to get dinner ready, take kids to activities, get them bathed and in bed, etc. and then finally find time to get everything else done for yourself, your cortisol levels start rising when they are supposed to decrease to ready your body for rest. If this happens, it makes it more difficult to get to sleep and stay asleep. See if you can shift some of your 'to-do' list to other times, or delegate them.

On top of it all, women especially, confuse sleepiness during the day with hunger and naturally go for carbs and sugar for energy, creating weight gain. We try to stuff so much into our days, thinking we can go with less sleep. Unfortunately, we can easily get our bodies messed up with issues like adrenal fatigue and weight gain, that our bodies forget how to create what is needed to get a good night's sleep.

Instead of trying to put Band-Aids on sleep problems with sleep aids, etc., it is important to address the causes for why our bodies can't seem to sleep, or stay asleep. Below is a list of ways to get a better night's rest by either getting rid of things that cause sleep disruption, or adding more relaxing rituals into your bedtime. It can be tough to change habits, but your body and everything around your life will drastically change for the better.

• Turn electronics off by 9pm and don't push yourself with extra activities.

- Decrease caffeine. There are people who can drink a cup at night and sleep right away and through the night. Others can drink a cup in the morning and because it might not effectively get through the system it creates sleep problems that night. We are all different and can develop sensitivities at different times in our lives. What you might have been able to ingest and digest before, you may not be able to do as effectively at this point. This can change again.

- If the mid-day slump hits, resist caffeine and sugar. Give your body what it really needs and take a short 10 min power nap, if you can. Don't trick the body out of the rest it needs as it will present its bill later with health issues.

- Create a whole bedtime ritual that is sacred to you. NO MATTER WHAT, protect this time as if your life depends on it, because it seriously does. Lack of sleep is a severe matter in our society. Take a bubble bath, read a book, turn your lights down sooner than later, use some of the amazing essential oils out there on the market.

- Keep all cell phones and screens out of the bedroom. Studies show that if you get up at night to pee it is highly likely that you will go check your phone and be sucked into social media land and emails, waking you and possibly causing anxiety that does not allow you to get back to sleep. If you use your phone as an alarm clock, get a traditional clock.

- Get horizontal before 10 pm. If you go past this time, you will get a second wind and have a hard time getting to sleep. If you are a self-professed night owl it is often because you have created a habit of going past this time. (The same goes for our kids). Try and flip it by getting to bed early and rising early to get everything done. You will wake more refreshed and able to accomplish SO much more during your day if you create this habit.

- Make sure your bedroom is completely dark and your bed is lush. Get the highest quality mattress and bed linens you can afford. you spend a huge chunk of time in bed, so make it worth it!

- Look up Yoga Nidra online. This is one of my FAVORITE relaxation techniques and I want you to start doing it. Look up breathing and relaxation recordings as they are also beneficial before you go to bed. Yoga Nidra is yogic sleep where 45 minutes equals about 3-4 hours of actual sleep! When I lead a Yoga Nidra workshop my participants always rave about how deep their sleep is that night! I hope to have some downloaded on my website, so make sure to check. Please try to do it at least 1-3 times a week or more, if needed.

- Magnesium is great as well (there is a product called Calm that works). Ask your doctor what she/he recommends and go from there.

- I also HIGHLY recommend getting your hormones checked. If they are off, everything else will be off and your sleep can be greatly affected. After our second child, my hormones went berserk and into a Peri-menopausal state. When I got them regulated by a specialist I was back in sleep heaven!

- Practice meditation to train your brain to focus on one thing, especially if your mind races at night.

- Decrease alcohol consumption as it will disrupt your sleep. It may help you get to sleep, but can bring you out of it as well later in the night.

- Eating protein instead of carbs at dinner has also been found to help with sleep.

- Also, halt any liquid consumption early in the evening to avoid waking in the night to pee. As mentioned before, keep a big glass of water by your bed to guzzle first thing in the morning to rehydrate your body.

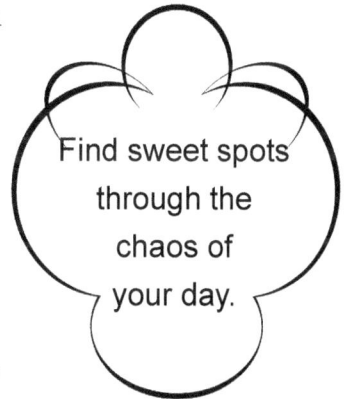

Find sweet spots through the chaos of your day.

All of this also goes for our kids. If you find your child has attention or behavioral issues, make sure they are getting the right type of sleep needed with the evening rituals to learn to slow down. They may simply be sleep deprived. We can so easily over-schedule them, so they can get over-stimulated and cannot unwind.

Note of awareness: Please give yourself time to see the results from creating a protected sacred habit around your sleep ritual. It took a lot to get you where you are presently, so it may take a while for your body and mind to learn to truly be able to chill out.

Please list some thoughts on your current state of sleep and what you will integrate to possibly improve it.

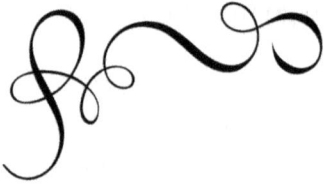

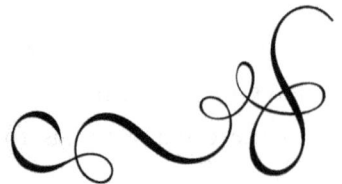

CHAPTER SEVENTEEN
Tone Up Your Mindset

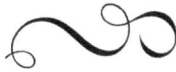

In closing, let's discuss our mindset, beliefs, and how we view our lives. EVERYTHING is affected by these, so it is important to understand that we have full control over them.

Remember that everything is a choice. I am not saying you stay out of reality and live in la-la land, but I will say that how you view things has a large impact on how you respond, or react, to life's dealings. You choose what you think and what and who you keep around, which defines your reality.

I could write an entire book on this topic, so I will save that for another time and not go into too much detail. But I will give you a few pointers and direction to go on for your own journey of exploration and growth.

Our bodies and minds consume everything that is around us. What we allow into our lives and what we focus on is what we will get more of. The more negative news you watch, the more negative of an outlook you will gain. Get the highlights of what is going on in the world, but don't get sucked into it. Find a news source that is all facts without emotions that can potentially ruffle your feathers.

The more gossip magazines you read the lower your vibration is to the great things in life. The more you hang with negative nellies and small-thinking people, the more you will become the same.

The opposite is also true. Through experience, I can attest to the "you are the average of the 5 people with whom you surround yourself" rule. When I started this journey toward really thriving in life, I looked at the people in my life. I started searching out people I admired. People who inspired me and who might mentor me, but also who I could bring value to with my gifts. By default, I began taking on the same qualities.

In so doing, you stop spending as much time with those who might pull you down. I am not saying to break up with anyone, or even have a specific conversation of why you might be less inclined to spend as much time as before (through doing this cleansing work, you might find you need to so to rid yourself of destructive relationships), but you naturally start gravitating toward those who are more aligned with your values. Remember your boundaries that you have created around your values and stick with them concerning everything you bring into your life.

Read books and magazines related to your dreams, your dream career, and your interests. These will broaden your mind and support your growth in these subjects.

Something that I have brought into my life that is now a non-negotiable is reading inspiring mindset books. These types of books have allowed me to think bigger, see what is possible and help me overcome self-limiting beliefs that were created and taken on throughout my life. I invite you to explore these types of books as they will open a whole broader world for you! They will help you address and let go of your own self-limiting beliefs. They help you release old stories you might have been telling yourself for decades, as well as the related self-sabotaging behaviors that keep you living smaller than you truly envision for yourself.

Some of my favorites that I have found as well as those recommended by my mentors and coaches, include:

- *The Magic of Thinking Big* by David Schwartz
- *Think and Grow Rich* by Napoleon Hill

- *The Science of Getting Rich* by Wallace Wattles
- *The Drama of the Gifted Child* by Alice Miller
- *Loving What Is* by Byron Katie
- *The Game of Life and How to Play It* by Florence Scovel Shinn
- *The Big Leap* by Gay Hendricks
- *The Dark Side of the Light Chasers* by Debbie Ford
- *Conscious Language* by Robert Tennyson Stevens
- *From Good To Great* by Jim Collins
- *The Alchemist* by Paulo Coehlo
- *Codependence No More* by Melody Beattie
- *The Energy Bus: 10 Rules to Fuel Your Life, Work and Team With Positive Energy* by Jon Gordon and Ken Blanchard

I invite you to seek some of these out and always be in the process of reading one, or more, like I do! You can get them on Kindle, for example, so they are all on one device, or get them in audible form to listen to while driving to make good use of your commutes.

Enjoy! Your mind is about to be blown (in a great way!)!

MINDSET THOUGHTS

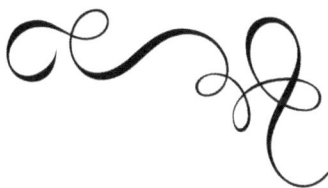

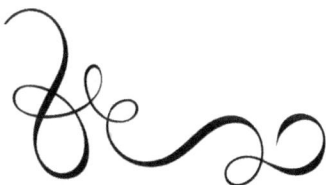

CONCLUSION

Keep Your Thriving Lifestyle Sustainable

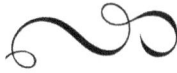

Whew! You did it! If you have followed the book and the steps herein, you have accomplished so much to help support yourself in getting off your Crazy-Busy Bus and into dynamic balance! Check it out!

You have:

- Determined and solidified your top priorities and created your Vision and Values Boards as well as a gratitude practice

- Attacked and cleared up your calendar to mirror and support your priorities

- Created boundaries around your time as well as what you say "yes" and "no" to

- Learned to delegate more effectively

- Toned up or de-cluttered and defined your surroundings

- Toned up your general affairs and nuisances

- Toned up and de-cluttered your food stash

- Learned various ways you can feed your amazing body

- Toned up your meal planning

- Toned up your food shopping

- Learned about eating patterns and reasons why you might hold on to your weight
- Toned up the body by finding joy in movement
- Learned various breathing techniques to combat stress
- Learned about mindfulness and meditation
- Toned up and committed to good relaxation and sleep
- Toned up your mindset so to bring growth and inspiration into your life

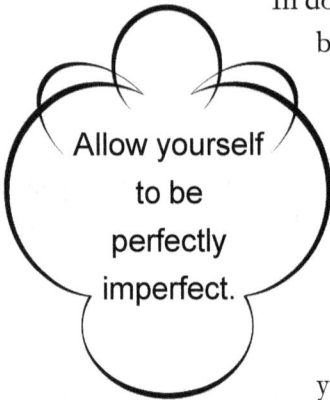

Allow yourself to be perfectly imperfect.

In doing so, you are much more able to create that dynamic balance we discussed earlier in the book. You have simplified and created the expansive systems for you to live in a more peaceful state and get off your Crazy-Busy Bus. You now can take mindful risks and go 'off balance' by pursuing goals related to your priorities, all the while supported by the self-care 'tethers' around the amount of time and action you take that will pull you back to center. When you have these controls of self-awareness, followed by actions that are in alignment with your priorities and values, **you run less of a risk of living a disjointed, anxiety-filled life, or otherwise known as burn out.**

Please know that all of this will take time, so give yourself grace to develop through the process. Allow for the changes to naturally occur over time. I assure you that you will gradually find yourself with so much more: more ease, more energy, more freedom, more joyful family time, and possibly more time in worship to your higher power, but with less irritability, stress and less weight.

Also, allow for those times when you completely still lose it. Those days are inevitable, but rest assured, you now have more tools to help you find your way back. Life is full of cycles for us to learn to ride. You are going to have times where things don't go your way. There will be days where the kids are constantly at each other's throats and you cannot calmly take a shower, or pee without an audience of little ones. These are times to embrace the chaos and witness the inherent beauty. **Breathe**. In the midst of all of it, create your moments of calm, or schedule times you can look forward to to help you through the tough times.

Common! You now totally know how to time out, tune in and tone up an incredible amount in your life and this is just the beginning. You have cleared out and created more support for yourself in your bus. You now can ease that foot off the pedal and determine what and how you want to drive because you are better equipped in your non-negotiable self-care and love! Because you now take care of yourself first and love yourself first, you can now love and serve with that which is overflowing from your reserves, rather than your 'fumes'.

In so doing, you are creating a life and lifestyle that are more sustainable, with less stress and more joy. You stop just functioning, but truly living. It is my hope that through all this you have learned that your self-care and self-preservation is non-negotiable. When you do, you will end up living a life that is richer with time to make more connections with others as well as with your internal wisdom. You end up living with fewer distractions because you are no longer addicted to your busy-ness with the need to constantly be doing something.

You have nothing to prove. **You are enough.** You now know how to take off your badge of honor of exhaustion and busy-ness! Remember that you are a human being. Not a human doing. Life is precious, so make it delicious!

Look at your Vision and Value Boards each day. Feed all aspects of yourself first by scheduling them in and treating them as you would any other appointment. When you do this, your overflow of energy and love will impact others, and they, in turn, will nourish you back. It's a win-win!

So, what are you waiting for? You are truly magnificent and you were placed here to shine that brilliance in your own unique way!

Go thrive again. And again. And Again.

THRIVE*Again*

*I don't want to get to the end of my life and find that I lived just the length of it.
I want to have lived the width as well.*
- Diane Ackerman

BONUS LIST

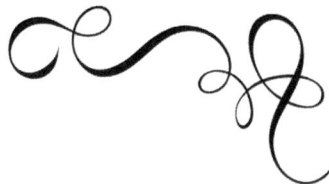

Here is a great list of random things you can do for ultimate self-care all wrapped up in a bow!

We are now all about self-care and preservation to THRIVE, so enjoy!

- Use any type of commute for good. Listen to audio books, pray, use it as a mindful transition to disengage between work and home, etc..

- Get silly when you are feeling stressed. Purposefully laugh, or growl as deeply as you can and you will feel the stress leave you more easily.

- Live moments of your life with total abandonment.

- Live in the moment.

- Remember that the world needs you and your full self at the table.

- Get over the need to 'do it all.'

- Schedule 'me' time and protect it like a mama bear.

- Schedule a quarterly get-away for yourself, even if it is at your home, or at a local hotel. Plan for some alone time to reflect on just YOU and your goals/desires.

- Find things that make your heart sing.

- Create specific morning and bedtime rituals that work for you.

- Kidnap your partner for lunch, or a get-away! Enough said!

- Play hooky and allow yourself to just do nothing for a day with no guilt.

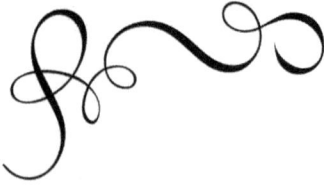

- Get in your favorite PJ's, socks and blanket and snuggle up OR dress up to the nines and spend the day at a luxury location!

- Tap into your spirituality, whatever that means to you.

- Sloooooooooow down.

- Breathe. Just breathe and be still.

- Build rejuvenation points into your day. Put on a timer if needed to stop what you are doing to consciously time out and breathe, rest, or or take a power nap!

- Allow yourself to be perfectly imperfect!

- Give yourself space between appointments so that you fully give yourself the needed breather to show up fully for the next thing.

- Time your pity parties. If something happens that you do not like, rant and rave and cry for 10 minutes and THEN BE DONE WITH IT!

- Plant a garden. This keeps you active, connected with nature and everyone involved will reap the benefits of your harvest.

- Belly laugh EVERY DAY!

- Don't forget to delegate!

- Put a timer on to get things done. Set a timer for 15 minutes to clear out a drawer, etc. This works wonders for kids as well!

- Throw the windows down in your car, blare the music and sing and dance to the toons!

- Plan a total get-away retreat for yourself once a year.

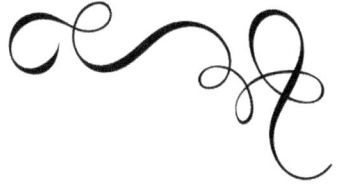

- Listen to music. DANCE! Go to a Zumba class, or a Tango bar and learn, or just jam in your house!

- Get out in nature. It is magical.

- End your day writing in your gratitude journal as well as your DONE/DON'T list. This one exercise can set your mind at ease and fill you with thanks as you drift off to sleep.

- Remember to keep your Vision and Value Boards visible for you to see every day.

- Create weekly regular rituals to support your life. For example, designate certain days to go grocery shopping, get the house cleaned, get laundry done, etc.

- Keep your weekends as clear as you can to help you rejuvenate. And keep one of those days dedicated to fully letting go for rest, worship, etc..

- Each Sunday sit down to plan out and structure your week (or whatever day works best for you).

- Keep your gasoline tank in your car at at least 1/2 at all times. When you do, you develop your self-care muscle and will never have the stress of running out of gas at the worst time possible

- Develop a creative outlet, whatever that may be. Take an art class. Pick up an instrument again. Learn to weld if that's your thing!

- Be OK with giving your kids more responsibility and hold them accountable to their actions. This lightens your load and gives them things to learn, do and feel empowered with a sense of pride.

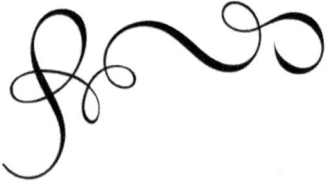

- Pay it forward in some way each day.

- Plan date nights! Again, enough said. :-)

- Respect other people's need for quiet alone time.

- Carve out time for your kids to have and embrace quiet alone time without electronics. They need the down time for their development and creativity.

- Carve out time for uninterrupted family time with fun, active activities. Do the same with your partner.

- Have a once a week NO-electronics day!

- Hire an organizer if you just cannot get your surroundings to a place that best supports you.

- Schedule fun and vacation in advance

- Practice good posture. This allows for better breathing as well as better functioning of all organs in the body. Your brain will get more oxygen and your body won't have to work so hard to live, which means you won't be as fatigued!

- Stop feeding your envy by comparing yourself to others. What is posted on Facebook is only the highlights of people's lives. You won't usually see the ugly.

- Make an effort to authentically smile often through the day.

- Shell out honest compliments to random strangers! Tell someone you love their outfit (if you do) as you walk past them.

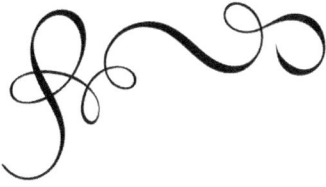

- If someone is throwing road rage at you, smile kindly at them and let them pass.

- Focus on being a blessing to another person while being a blessing to yourself first.

- Focus on the goodness inside others rather than finding their flaws. This starts with yourself and toward yourself!

- Fears come from the unknown. Getting a better understanding of a situation will lessen your fear.

- Develop trust in yourself and your abilities through little successes.

- Get all of your doctor appointments scheduled when needed.

- Get your car serviced regularly.

- Have an emergency fund for the unexpected times. Feeling secure financially can make all the difference on your stress levels and health.

- Put yourself on a social media and news channel detox.

- Be aware of what distracts you and lessen those. Nip them in the bud.

- Buy fresh flowers on a regular basis.

- Take a nap when you can, even if for 10 minutes.

- Keep the number of choices you have to make each day to a minimum. There's nothing worse than a 10-page menu at a restaurant.

- Create an 'hour of power', or 'day of Awesome Get-it-Done-ness'! This is a period completely dedicated to getting something or things done with intense focus.

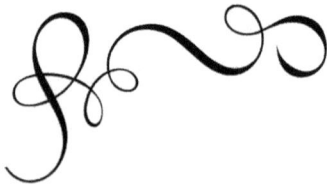

- Try being a little early to everything.

- Set intentions for the day, week, month, year and stick with the actions that support those.

- Do one thing that scares you on a regular basis. Step outside your comfort zone. You'd be surprised what might happen.

- Most importantly, as shown through this whole book, make taking care of #1 a first priority. Only then can you help others.

In closing, I leave you with one of my favorite prayers to say concerning living life, and I hope you will benefit from it as much as I do:

God, use me. Use me.
Use this life. I don't know what the future
holds for me, but I know that there is a vision for my life that is greater
than my imagination.
Use me. Use me.
What will You have me do?
-Oprah

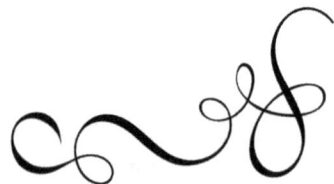

For speaking engagements, please write to:

eli@elidemoraes.com

www.Facebook.com/elizabethelidemoraes

www.Instagram.com/elidemoraes

www.Pinterest.com/elidemoraes

www.YouTube.com/elidemoraes

ABOUT THE AUTHOR
Eli de Moraes, M.A., M.F.A., R.Y.T.

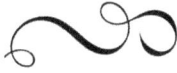

www.ElideMoraes.com

Eli comes to you with decades of entrepreneurial experience in the health and fitness industries. She is an accomplished former international professional dancer with multiple Master degrees, a Pilates and yoga teacher, and a Transformational Health and Lifestyle Coach.

After finding herself wrapped in a blanket on the ground in her backyard during a nervous breakdown because of too many stressors pulling on her, she knew she had to make a change. Life as she knew it was not sustainable. She pulled herself up, finally realizing that her actions were completely out of balance in relation to her priorities. She had become addicted to the busy-ness of life, and, as a result, had become everything to everyone and couldn't let go of the choke-hold she had placed on her life. She wore her busy-ness and exhaustion as a badge of honor, but that approach no longer served her.

As a Transformational Health and Lifestyle Coach, she is passionate about empowering other women across the globe, by encouraging them to stop living in overwhelm and to fully live and express themselves on their terms. This is done with setting firm priorities and acting upon those, surrounded by boundaries of simple, yet profound, stress prevention methods. These are then supported by stress management tools for when the everyday realities pull.

With a huge porch swing, she currently lives in the Dallas area with her husband and two daughters across the street from a farmers market. She hosts a monthly local TV show about the market, the community gardens, & her city's sustainability efforts. In addition to seeing her Coaching clients, she is passionate about teaching yoga and Pilates to provide a holistic approach to the whole person.

Her mantra: Life is too long to live in agony and too short to waste away, so let's go and **THRIVE**!

THRIVEAgain

Gratitude Journal

&

DONE/DON'T List

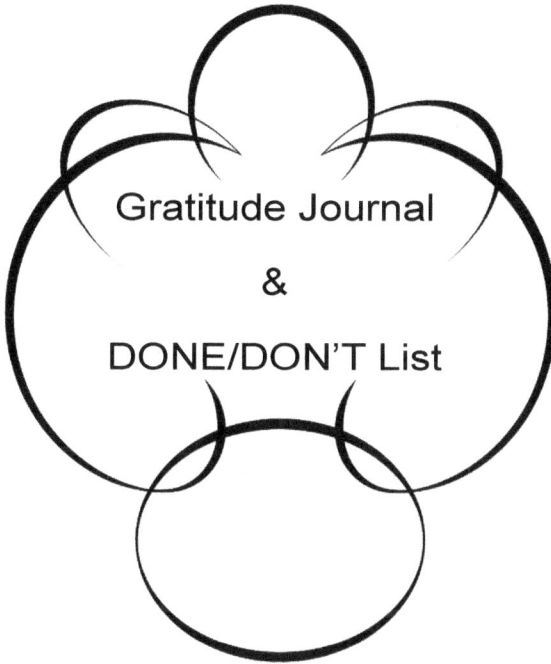

This is your sacred place to write out your daily points of gratitude as well as what you accomplished today. You may also write reminders of what you will not do.

It is purposefully left open so that you can fill it in as you see fit.

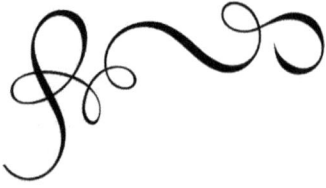

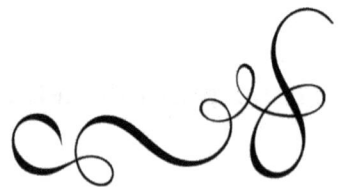

Eli de Moraes

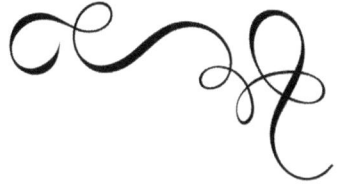

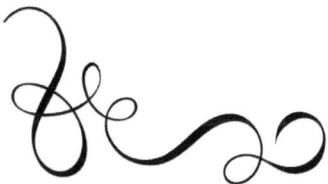

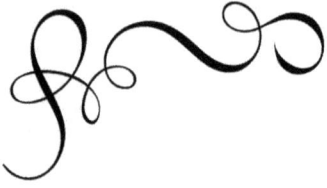

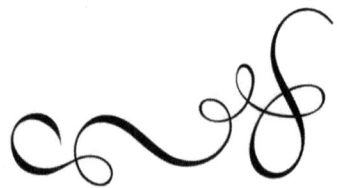

Eli de Moraes

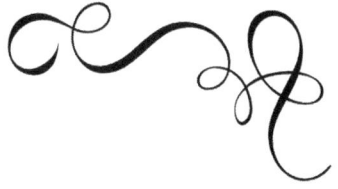

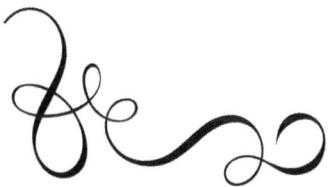

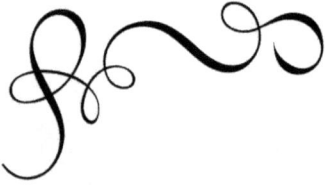

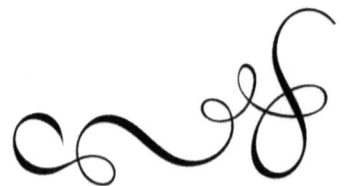

Eli de Moraes

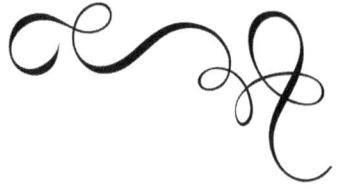

123

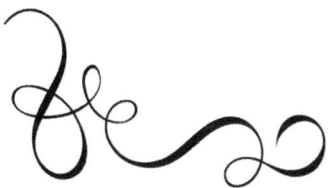

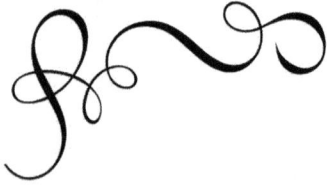

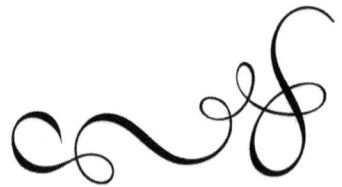

Eli de Moraes

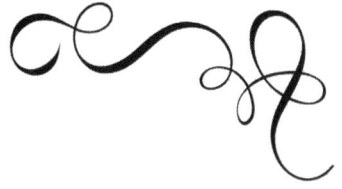

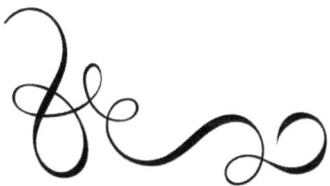

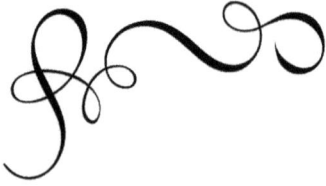

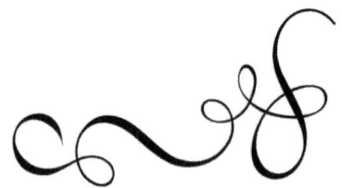

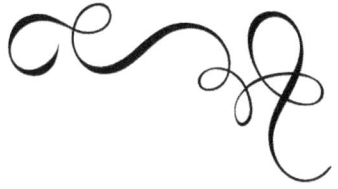

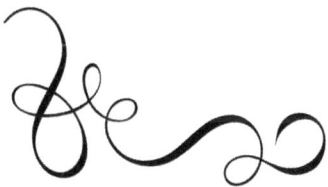

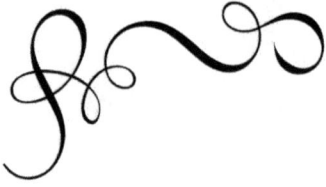

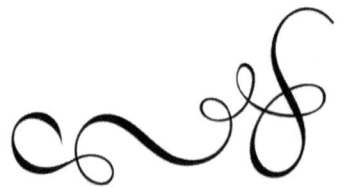

Eli de Moraes

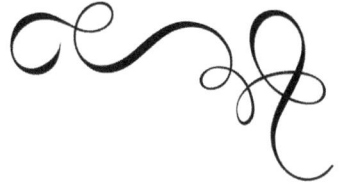

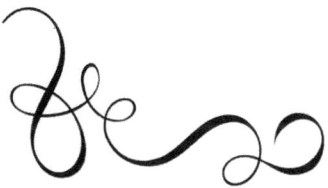

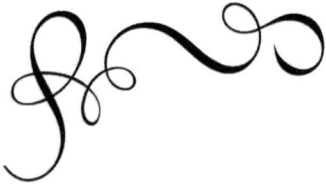

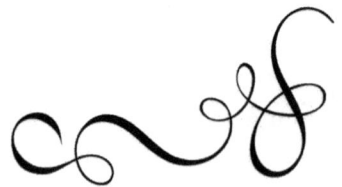

Eli de Moraes

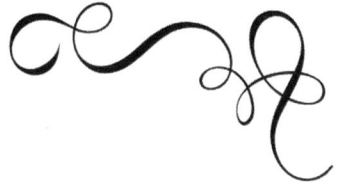

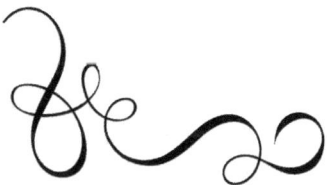

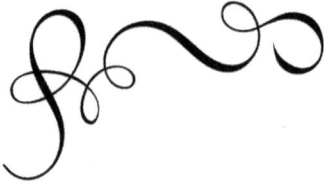

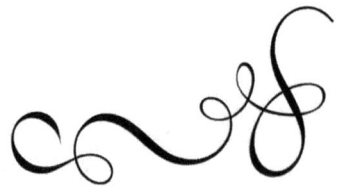

Eli de Moraes

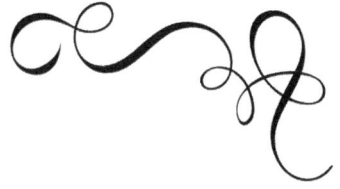

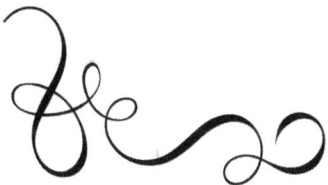

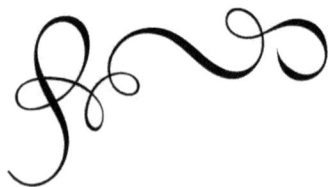

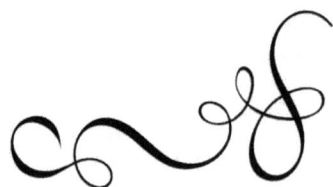

Eli de Moraes

135

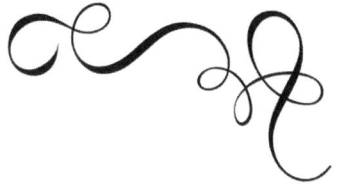

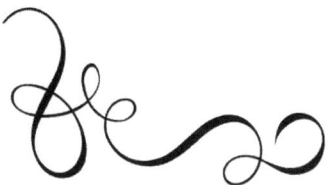

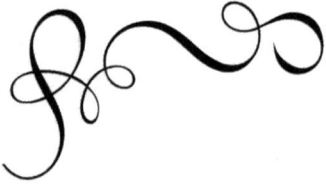

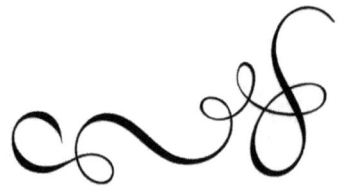

Eli de Moraes

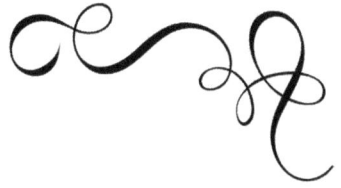

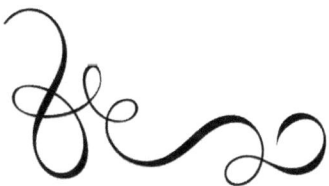

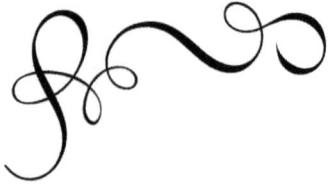

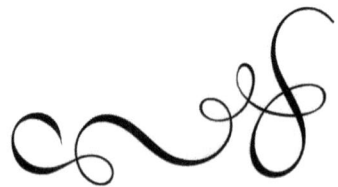

Eli de Moraes

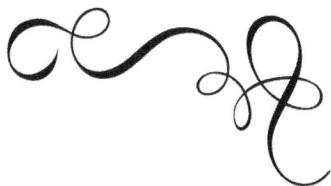

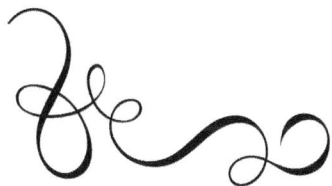

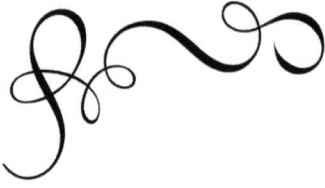

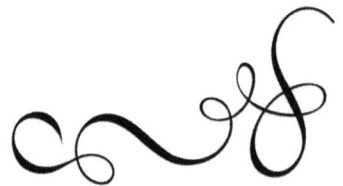

Eli de Moraes

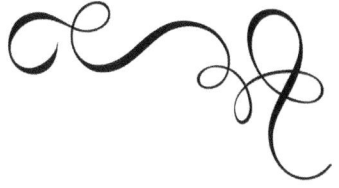

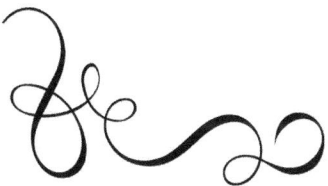

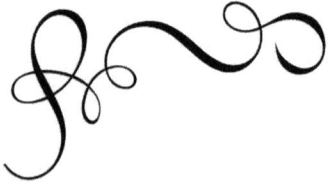

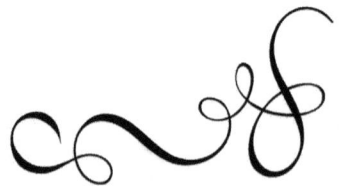

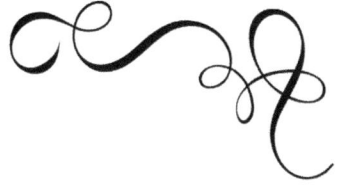

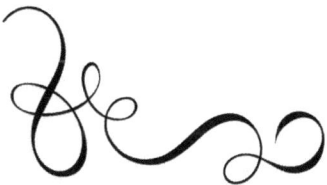

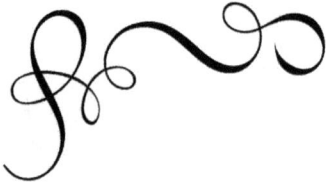

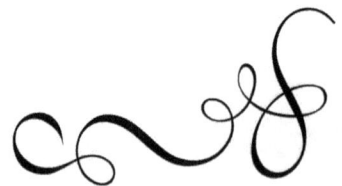

Eli de Moraes

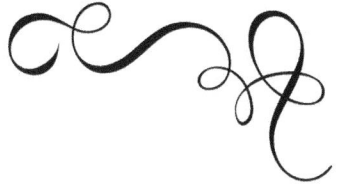

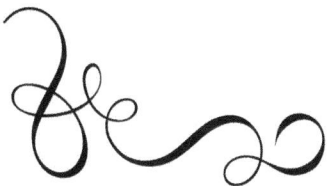

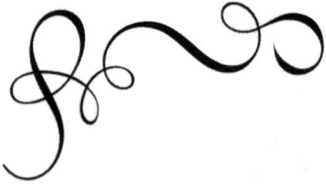

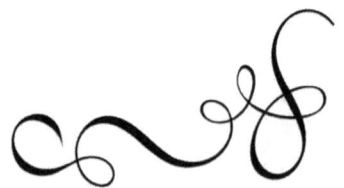

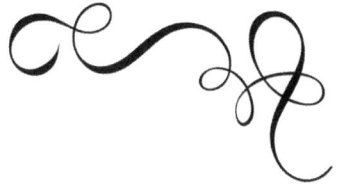

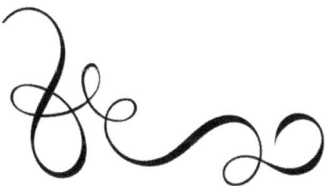

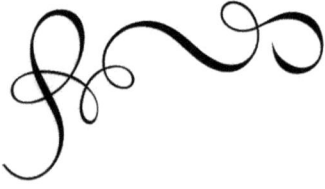

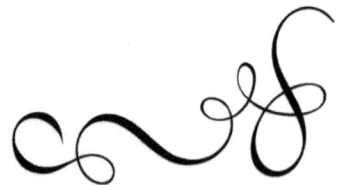

Eli de Moraes

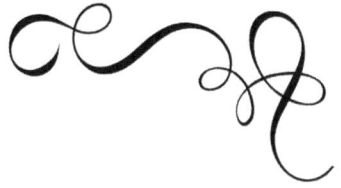

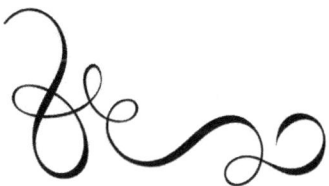

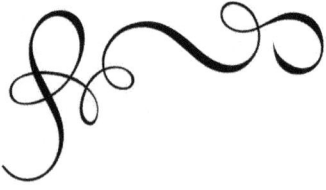

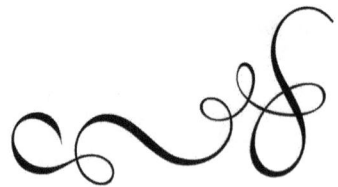

Eli de Moraes

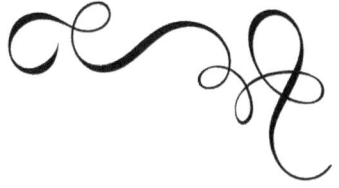

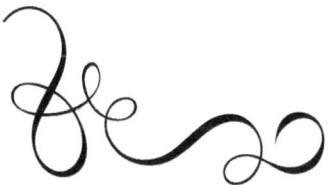

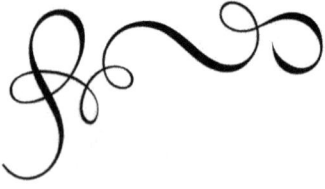

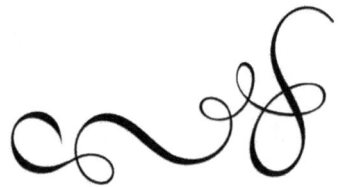

Eli de Moraes

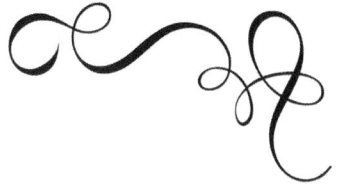

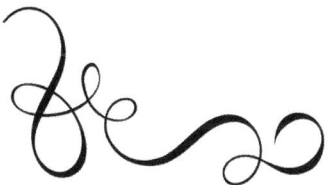

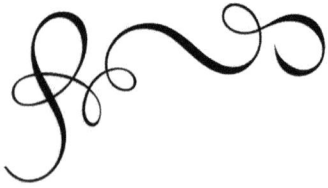

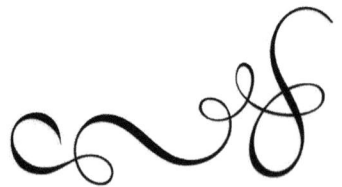

Eli de Moraes

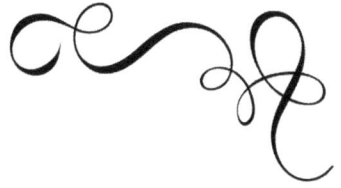

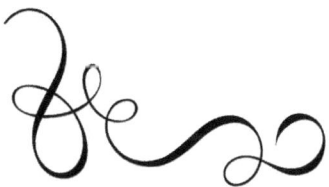

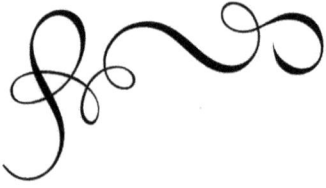

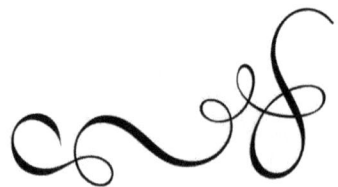

Eli de Moraes

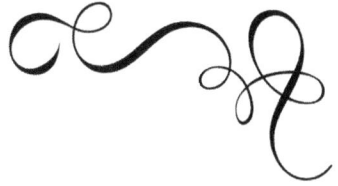

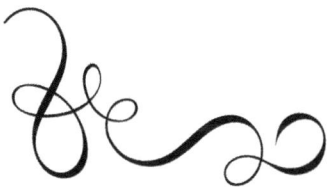

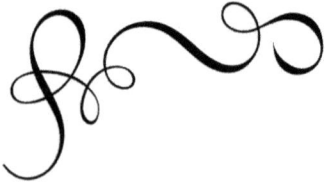

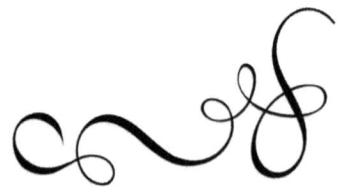

Eli de Moraes

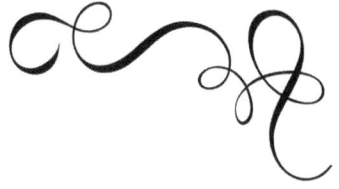

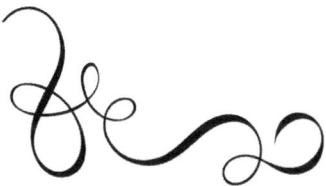

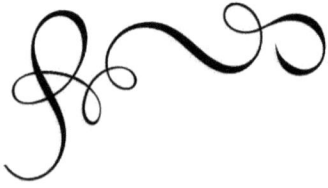

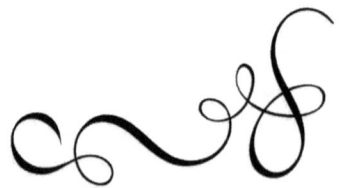

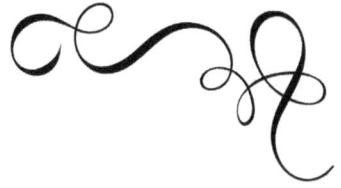

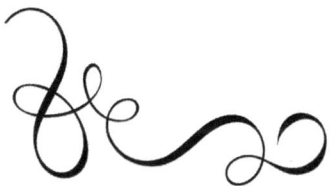

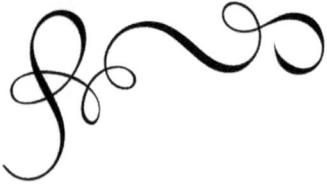

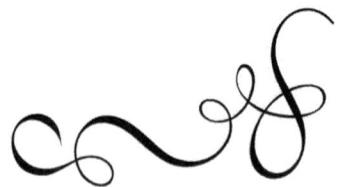

Eli de Moraes

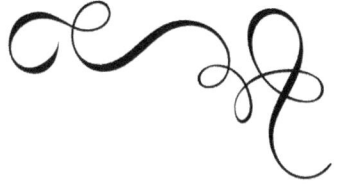

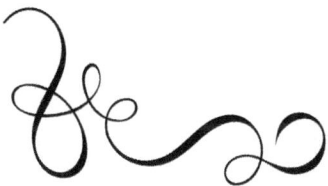

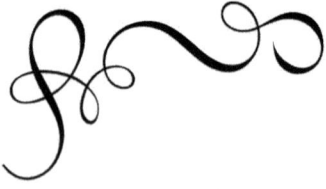

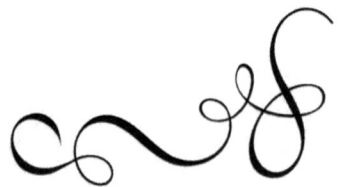

Eli de Moraes

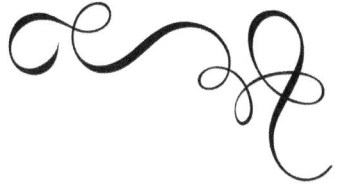

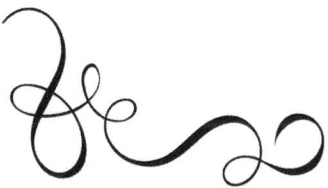

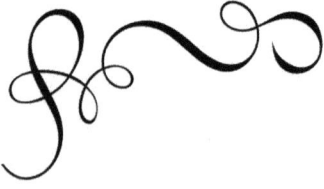

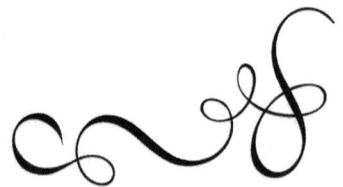

Eli de Moraes

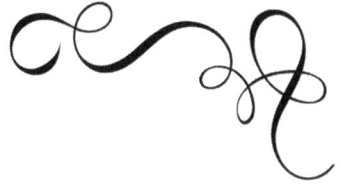

May you be abundantly blessed!

oxox,

Eli

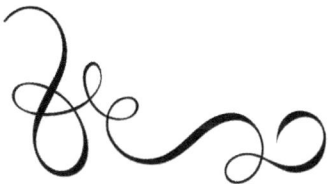

www.ingramcontent.com/pod-product-compliance
Lightning Source LLC
Chambersburg PA
CBHW070839300326
41935CB00038B/1149